WHO'S AFRAID OF THE TEDDY BEAR'S PICNIC
(A STORY OF SEXUAL ABUSE AND RECOVERY THROUGH PSYCHOTHERAPY)

BY

PAM SMART

All rights reserved, no part of this publication may be reproduced by any means, electronic, mechanical, or photocopying, documentary, film, or otherwise without prior permission of the publisher.

Published by:
Chipmunkapublishing
PO Box 6872
Brentwood
Essex
CM13 1ZT
United Kingdom

http://www.chipmunkapublishing.com

Copyright © 2006 Pam Smart

ISBN 978 1 84747 026 3

The development of this book was made possible by a grant from The Arts Council, London.

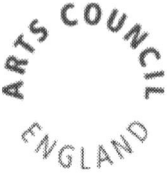

Foreword

I would like to introduce you to Pam. She is a mother and a grandmother. She works as a psychotherapist and for many years she worked as a social worker, working with people with learning difficulties.

Life for Pam now is fulfilled and mainly happy. It wasn't always this way. It took courage and determination for Pam to work through and understand her turbulent and terrifying childhood.

CHAPTER ONE

I feel terrified.
"I have made a most dreadful mistake."
I look around our three-bedroom council flat that is situated on the fifth floor.
"Where are the children going to play? There is no garden and they can't possibly go down five flights of stairs to play in the courtyard on their own."
Panic sweeps over me.
"What have I done?"
The room is swaying around me; cracks appear in the wall, the building is going to collapse. I can't hear what Simon, or other people are saying to me, everything and everyone is moving in slow motion.
"I must run; I have to get out of this flat."
I am on the street and the pavement has developed huge chasms. An earthquake is happening, but it is only happening to me, other people don't seem to notice.
I do not know how but I have found myself at the office of the social services. The duty social worker Maria is talking to me. I think that we are talking about the possibility of a transfer to another flat that would be lower than the fifth floor. Maria says that she will come and visit my family and me.
I am at King's Cross station. I am ready to throw myself under a train. A Policewoman stops me just as I reach the platform, I hit out and try to run, she restrains me and I am taken into an office where there are more police. I am not safe; I cry out that I need to get back to the children's home; I have got to get back to Mummy Robins, my housemother.

I wake up a week later in Friern Barnet psychiatric hospital. I have been sectioned under the Mental Health Act and Simon, my husband, has signed an authorisation form giving them permission to give me Electro Convulsive Therapy (E.C.T.). I am a mess, everything is a total haze, and I am told that Simon's parents are looking after our children, Jay and Beth. Maria, the duty social worker, comes to visit me in the hospital. She is a young woman, who is about the same age as me. She is happy to sit and talk to me. She tells me in a foreign accent: "I am your allocated social worker and I will be visiting you at your home when you leave hospital."

She adds that I can also see her at her office if I need to. I stay in the psychiatric hospital for two or three months, I have five or six whacks of E.C.T. and they also give me large doses of Largactyl. When I leave hospital I feel like a walking zombie.

Whilst I was in hospital, social services had us moved, so I arrived home to a new flat on a small estate just off the Holloway road. We live on the first floor and Jay and Beth can continue to attend the school that they had started whilst I was away. I am required to continue to go back to see the psychiatrist in her outpatients' clinic. I go, but I say nothing. I stare out of the window as scenes from my childhood flash through my mind.

I begin to turn up unannounced at Maria's office, which is in a basement of an old derelict church in Market Road about ten minutes walk from where I am living with Simon and our children. Maria is Dutch, she doesn't look like an official person, she dresses in a pair of jeans and a top, her hair is long and curly and it falls loosely around her shoulders. Maria never turns me away or makes a fuss about seeing me on spec. If she has to go out she says, "Pam I have to go out for a while. Julia is making you a cup of coffee and I will be back." Julia, the receptionist, talks to me in between answering the phone and dealing with visitors. It is almost as if Maria senses that I need to be kept safe until she gets back to the office. I find Maria easy to talk to and I begin to tell her about the children's home, how I loved it there, and I also find myself telling her about the sexual abuse, by Uncle Harry.

During my teens I had been hospitalised. I was given drugs, put in a hospital cell and given E.C.T. My mother's voice comes into my head, "You must not tell." Here I am telling Maria. She refers me to a psychiatric day centre. The day centre staff encourage me to talk to them about things that bother me, always things from the past. I do not have enough words and I start to act out on a large scale, I am very self-destructive. On one occasion I cut myself so badly on my arms and stomach that the medical staff called the police because they thought the injuries so severe that they could not be self-inflicted. I never feel any pain nor do I know why I am doing it. I go into a dreamlike state where I feel compelled to go and steal the razor blades and cut myself, I am also drinking and smashing windows, either in our flat or in the hospital. One of my workers from the day centre takes me across the road to some derelict buildings and encourages me to vent my feelings by smashing glass. He says, "This is better than cutting yourself Pam."

I am not conscious of feeling anything, but I don't cut myself this time.

My severe acting out continues over a period of eighteen months. There are several occasions when I am sectioned and I spend time in hospital. At these times Jay and Beth go into care, because Simon's parents say that they cannot look after them. This makes me feel worse, I feel that I am a bad mother, useless and unworthy.

One time I am given hospital leave to visit Jay and Beth in the children's home. I sit on the bus approaching the traffic lights and it goes through my mind if the lights turn red I won't cut myself, but if they turn green then I will. I do not make the visit to my children on this occasion.

Maria and Pat, a member of the day centre staff, are very supportive. They accompany me to the hospital for stitches many times and let me talk at great length. I go over the same thing over and over again, the sexual and physical abuse by Uncle Harry. I also tell them about how what had started out as sexual games with my brothers, in the children's home, turned into abuse by the time we had left care. Over a period of time I tell Pat, Maria and other day centre staff what I know of the story of my life at this time

ABANDONED BABY
CHAPTER TWO

A picture comes to mind. Nanny Donnelly is drinking a cup of tea and sharing a packet of jam tarts with me. I am about eight years old. She looks serene as a sunbeam comes through the lace curtains and catches her silver hair in the light. She is a small, well-dressed elderly woman. She tells me, "You were about six months old when you went into care, and by two and a half you became very ill. Pam, you were such a poor little thing, you lay in your cot refusing to eat or have anything to do with anyone. You just turned your back and stared into space. You were wasting away. I insisted that you went to live in the Hollies with your brothers."
I look around Nanny Donnelly's room. I don't ask any questions. I know not to ask, just accept what she says and keep quiet.

A different image comes to mind. The Hollies, a children's home in Sidcup Kent, is a grand, palatial group of houses set in open park land, built in Victorian times. Although all the houses are referred to as cottages, there is nothing of the cottage about them. They are huge and imposing. The complex includes its own laundry and kitchens. The food is cooked in the main kitchen, and then delivered to the various cottages. There is a swimming pool and I learn how to swim by the age of three although I am backward in all other areas of development. There is a tree house and a huge play park with a climbing frame, sand pit, cricket pitch and lots of green areas with big old trees. I don't wear or have my own clothes, we wear underwear and dresses, or trousers for the boys, that are our size and came from the main store.

My mind moves on again. I can see lots of children. I am being pushed in a pushchair. I can see lots of big children; I am like a toy for them, a dolly in a pram. I am clutching a baby's feeding bottle and I can feel my fingers holding it very tightly. For some reason I cannot walk. I watch the bigger children playing; they are all talking at once, jumping up and down with a rope. They seem happy.

Interestingly I grow up to be an observer of others.

I am to be in Rose Cottage with Mummy Robins, the housemother. Joe and Dennis are already in another cottage with a different housemother. I think I am the baby of the house and Mummy Robins favours me. She is a small woman, slim, no taller than five feet, she is always neatly groomed and her short neat hair is permed into waves, so that it sweeps backwards off of her face. She has protruding front teeth, which sometimes makes it difficult to understand some of her words. My brother Joe says that she is an odd looking woman, but to me she is beautiful.

Mummy Robins is like my mother and I love to sneak into her bedroom in the middle of the night. I do not remember when this started. Sometimes I wake up feeling scared in the middle of the night. Half asleep, I walk dreamily down the long corridor and down a flight of stairs. I turn the huge door-knob and slowly open the door to Mummy Robins bedroom, and stand by the side of her bed. She sits up in her bed and reaches for the light switch on the wall.
"Pam, it's you. What's wrong? Can't you sleep?"
She pulls back the covers of the bed. Pats the bed and says, "Come on then, hop in."
I feel warm and safe. I snuggle down to sleep.

I wake up the next morning and Mummy Robins is already up and dressed.

"Come on, sleepy head, up and get dressed."

She shouts to Nancy, one of the older girls:

"Nancy, have you finished dressing Barry? Well, come and help with Pam."

Nancy roughly pulls me from the bed and leads me by the hand into a big bathroom where other kids are getting washed and dressed. She quickly pulls my nighty over my head, washes my face and dresses me in the same summer dress that I wore yesterday. She hurriedly brushes my hair, missing the back of my head completely. Without speaking to me or looking at me Nancy again takes my hand and half pulls me along the corridor, down a flight of stairs to the huge table where we eat our breakfast

I look at all the other children sitting up at the table and I attempt to join them by climbing onto an empty chair. Carol, another older child, helps me up by yanking me up under my arm onto the chair. The room is silent; no one talks when we are up at the table. Eggs and a plateful of bread that are cut into quarters are passed around the table in an orderly fashion. It's not long before all the food has been eaten and a hubbub of noise fills the room. I remain sitting and I watch the older kids clear the table while the younger ones struggle to put their coats on. They are all soon in a straight line outside Rose cottage waiting to be taken to school. I spend a long day at home with Mummy Robins. Although I can now walk, my speech isn't forthcoming. I watch what's going on around me, in my silent world, rather than joining in. I remain at the dining room table and wait. The other children are not allowed to do this. The other children in the house are jealous of the attention I get from Mummy Robins, and I am frequently smacked and punished by the member of staff in charge when Mummy Robins is on holiday or has a day off.

There is a new girl in Rose cottage and her name is Ruthy. Ruthy and I become playmates, the other children are older and during the day they are at school. Ruthy and I are too young for school, so we stay at the children's home. Ruthy is a little black girl. She chatters away to me and never seems to mind that I don't respond to her. Ruthy puts me in my pushchair and attempts to wheel me around the house, her being the grown up and me being the child.

Over the weeks I gradually begin to join in with Ruthy's games, we sleep in the same room, have our baths together and play with each other all day. It is a sad day for me when Ruthy leaves the Hollies. I watch in stunned silence as a smiling Ruthy is dressed in a smart set of clothes and a little bag is packed for her. Then these strange people, who I have never seen before, walk along the path towards the main gate with Ruthy. Ruthy disappears out of my sight. Mummy Robins tells me that the nice couple have chosen her. It seems as if you have to be very special to be chosen. I wonder if anyone will choose me.

I begin to get to know my brothers. I adore Joe, Dennis seems weak, and I think that he is a crybaby. Dennis is punished and treated very badly by his housemother, who tells us, "You are lucky to be here. Other people have to pay for your keep and you should be grateful for what you have: good food and a nice place to live."
"It is a hard world out there and you have got to learn to toughen up."
She will not tolerate Dennis or any other child crying or making a fuss. When I go for tea with Joe and Dennis at their house, Dennis is slow at eating his kippers; he doesn't like fish and he sits at the table staring at his plate.
Miss Harris, his housemother, demands that he finishes eating saying, "You are an ungrateful boy."

She asks him, "Do you want your pudding, child?"
Dennis says in a small voice, "Yes please."
She pours the custard over his fish and force-feeds him. None of us children flinch or say a word, that's how it is. To us her behaviour is normal. Any other member of staff would do the same thing.

It's Dennis's birthday, and I have brought him some sweets out of my one penny a week pocket money. Joe and Dennis are standing near my cottage looking up the path to the big main gate. They are dressed in short trousers with bib and brace. Whilst we all have blue eyes, Dennis has short blond curly hair and Joe's is dark and straight. My short blond curly hair is held in place with a ribbon. I think to myself this must mean that the staff are expecting someone to visit us. Dennis is convinced that our mother is coming to visit him. She does not come and Dennis doesn't dare cry, so he just stands there and messes and pees into his pants. To wet your pants or your bed is a sign of weakness and Dennis is severely punished by his housemother.

Joe tells me that I should love my real mother whoever she might be. When my mother's boyfriend, Uncle Harry, whom I must know already, introduces me to her, it is a bright summer day and this huge man gently pushes me towards this woman. He says, as he pushes me towards her, "Go on, it's your mum. Say hello to your mum."
I am bemused. I don't know her. She stands there, dressed in a light summer coat, and her long hair, which is held in a bun, is the same colour as Joe's. I feel confused because I have a mum, Mummy Robins.

My mother starts to visit regularly and after a while takes us home for some weekends. My mother lives with Uncle Harry and his mother. I cling to Mummy Robins and refuse to go. My mother and Uncle Harry are furious with Mummy Robins. They say that she spoils me. Mummy Robins, all of a sudden, becomes very distant and cold.

She says, "You must not ask me for a cuddle, you are bigger now and from now on I have to treat you like the other children."

Miss Harris, my brother's housemother, tells my mother and Uncle Harry that I should be transferred to her house and she will soon teach me how to behave properly.

"What does Mummy Robins mean? What have I done wrong?"

I feel alone and confused. A feeling of shame sweeps over me as the other children taunt me.

"You're not the favourite one now, are you? You're not so bloody special after all. She isn't going to stand up for you or take your side anymore, is she? So you better watch out, spoilt brat."

My best friend at the children's home is Michael. Michael doesn't shout at me like the other kids, instead, like my brothers, he protects me and if I can, I look after Michael. Michael lives in the same house as me, and is Nancy's younger brother, although he is a bit older than me. He has lots of other brothers and sisters. Michael's mum died and his father abandoned all eight of his children and went back to live in Ireland. Mummy Robins doesn't like Michael. She picks on him and he is punished almost daily. One of the things that Michael gets punished for is for wetting his bed.

One morning when Michael comes into my dormitory he tells me in a panicky, shaky voice, "I've wet my bed again, Pam."

His light brown hair stands up on end and his brown eyes are full of fear. It isn't morning and finding clean sheets from the linen cupboard and putting the wet sheets into the

big brown wicker basket in the dawn light is a hopeless task.
We are caught by Nancy, who wakes up and says, in a spiteful voice, "I'm going to tell on you!"
The wet sheet is rubbed into Michael's face and we both spend the day sitting on the floor, in the corner of the dining room.

Mummy Robins tells me that my mother and Uncle Harry are coming to collect me for the weekend; I don't want to go with them. After breakfast I hide in the woods. The woods are across the road from Rose cottage and stretch to the big main gate. The trees are good friends of mine; their leaves make patterns for me as the sunlight shines through their crowns. This is a very special and safe space and I sit and daydream for hours. I dream of being chosen, and of being taken away from this place. I daydream about the time when Mummy Robins took me to her mother's house for the day.

We go on a very long bus ride and as we walk down the street Mummy Robins holds my hand tightly and I walk along the pavement beside her. I feel so happy. When we reach a little house, Mummy Robins looks at me and reminds me that I have to be good.

She says, "My mother is a very old lady and doesn't like a lot of noise, sit still and don't fidget and do not touch anything."

A very old lady opens the door and Mummy Robins guides me into a small room. I am sat on a big padded armchair; my feet only just reach the end of the seat. I look around the room in amazement. The room is full of pretty objects and photographs that are on the mantelshelf and on small tables. The sunlight shines through the net curtains and streams through the window onto many of the pretty objects. The old lady gives me a piece of cake on a small plate.

She smiles at me and says, "Don't make a mess, will you?"

I'm hungry and cold; the sun isn't shinning through the trees any longer. Time has passed, it is now teatime. I come out from the woods and return to Rose cottage, I shiver with fear and cold. I know that I will be punished. I am told that I need to think very carefully about being disobedient in future.

I spend lots of time during the day on my own or with my brothers. I love to be with them.
Joe says to me, "You must be strong, Pamela, don't ever cry, don't let '**THEM**' see that you are scared of them."
I know that Joe is right; the kids who are seen as weak and cry are punished without mercy. We are expected to be strong and grateful.

I think that this is when the sexual games start with Joe and Dennis. We would have a peeing contest, to see which one of us could get their pee to travel the furthest. We touch and stroke each other's bodies and genitals. I felt a warm tingling running through my body. I feel loved and wanted. Of course we are all very careful not to get caught.

When I am old enough I go to the local school, all the kids walk to school at the same time in crocodile fashion. We walk in twos, holding onto the hand of the child next to us; I don't know why but I am dropped off first, probably because I am the youngest. I don't seem to make friends with the other kids at school; they come from real families. We, the kids from the home, are known as the 'Gutter snipes' and we are to be avoided. It doesn't matter that I am simple or slow at learning how to read and write; to fail is expected by the teachers and the staff from the Hollies.

I hate going to school. I feel out of my depth and that I don't belong here. I could hear what the parents of other children say to them.

"Stay away from her, she is rough and is trouble."

I stand alone in the playground, staring at the floor, whilst the other kids are playing and having fun. If I get in their way, they push and shove me and spit at my feet, saying, "Scum, what are you doing here?"

Once I start school, I go home every four or five weeks for the weekend. I stay with my mother and Uncle Harry at Nanny Donnelly's house; I don't know where Joe and Dennis stay. I hate it and I spend most of my time sitting under the dining room table rocking.

Nanny Donnelly is a small old woman with short grey hair; she has fine features and bright blue eyes. She dresses very smartly and is a bundle of energy. Nanny Donnelly has three rooms in a house, which she shares with another family; there is the kitchen come sitting room and two bedrooms. These rooms are on the top floor. There is spotlessly clean dark lino on the floor, with one or two rugs. We sit at a large dining table for our meals and in the evening Nanny Donnelly and Uncle Harry sit in two old armchairs. There is a big ceramic sink, which is used for the washing-up, washing clothes and bathing. A small white cooker also lives in this room, which isn't that big. Both families share the outside toilet.

The woman who occupies the ground floor and the first floor has about seven children. The steps, which lead to the street, are always cluttered with children sitting on them. There is a constant din with the kids playing in the street with other children from the area and children running in and out of the house and up and down the bare stairway.

The woman shouts out, "Make you're bloody mind up, either come in or stay outside, and don't you dare wake your father up."

I never see their father in all the times that I stay at Nanny Donnelly's house.

When I get a little older, Nanny Donnelly sends me to the corner shop, "Ask Ethel for five weights, a bottle of stout and a packet of jam tarts. Tell her to put it on my slate and I will pay for it at the end of the week."

I enjoy running this errand for Nanny Donnelly; I run along Durham Road, there aren't many cars, just lots of children playing in the street. I feel as if I belong here, on this street, the children ask me if I want to join in their game, and it seems that Nanny Donnelly likes having me to stay.

My mother's mother has some land in Kent. Grandmother Samuels, I am told, is a wealthy Jewish woman, although she does not practice the Jewish faith. The camp, as it is called, is down a quiet country lane in Romford. There are several chalets, one big one, which is where the food is cooked and where we eat, then lots of smaller chalets, which are used as bedrooms. My mother and Uncle Harry take Joe, Dennis and me there. We spend one or two weeks during the summer. There is always lots of work to do: cutting very long grass, painting and other repair jobs. I do not do that many chores, because I am seen as too little, but the boys are put to work.

My job is to sleep in the same chalet as Grandma Samuels, who is a very, very old lady. She is a large lady who doesn't say very much to me, in fact she doesn't say very much to anyone, just nudges him or her out of her way with her walking stick, with a grunt of, "Move, move out of my way."

"Ring the bell if she is sick during the night," my mother says.

There always seems to be a damp smell in all the chalets, as well as the smell of paraffin from the paraffin oil lamps and the aroma of Uncle Harry's pungent cigarettes. It feels as if he is always present watching me and will know what I am doing or thinking. Once my mother has settled Grandma Samuels into bed, the oil lamp is blown out and we are left in the darkness, where I listen to her breathing and wonder if she is going to die.

Uncle Harry does not like my Grandma Samuels or other members of my mother's family; the feeling seems to be mutual, as my mother's brothers and sisters mainly stay away from our family. My mother tells me that two of her sisters, Aunty Vi and Aunty Rachel, looked after my brothers when she was ill in hospital. She says that they couldn't look after me as well and that her sister Kitty would only take me if my mother let her adopt me. I have day dreamed about being adopted for years, as far back as I can remember. I know that my mother doesn't love me.

She says, in a sullen blaming voice, "It was your fault that I didn't visit you in the nursery because when I visited you, you would look away from me. I got so upset when you rejected me, that I had to stay away. I couldn't bear to see you turn away from me, it was better that I stayed away. You did the same thing to me when I first came to see you at the children's home. You pushed me away, you wanted to stay with Miss Robins, so don't you try and make out that it was my doing."

I felt confused and to blame, yet at the same time I was scared of being with my mother who couldn't bear to have me near to her.

Whilst we were at the camp my mother would push me towards Uncle Harry. She would say, "Go and sit on Uncle Harry's lap."

Uncle Harry is a huge man, over six feet tall and weighs about twenty-six stone. He has thinning hair and looks much older than my mother. He is lying on a sun lounger and my mother pushes me towards him. He puts his massive hands under my tiny elbows and lifts me up to rest on his huge paunch. He is not wearing a top and his trousers are undone. He strokes my hair then tickles me under my arms, and then my tummy and he keeps tickling me until he reaches the tops of my legs. He continues to tickle, but hard, and then he pinches the inside of my thighs. I can't stop myself from laughing and crying at the same time.

I say, "No more, No more!" Then I wet myself.

He throws me off of him slapping my bottom, saying to my mother, "Get her washed and changed, she is a filthy little bitch."

It is a hot summer day, I am sitting daydreaming, which is what I seem to do a lot, and I am wearing a pair of shorts but no top, because it is such a very hot day. I sat there stroking my chest. He comes up behind me and pulls me by my hair, bends me over and canes me.

He says in front of my mother and the boys, "She is a filthy little slag and she must wear a top at all times."

I don't cry. I just go inside myself. I haven't got a clue what I have done wrong.

Caning becomes a regular punishment for my brothers and me, for any minor transgression of Uncle Harry's rules.

The last summer holiday that we spend at the camp, Grandmother Samuels dies. On the day of the funeral, Joe, Dennis and myself are left alone at the camp while my mother and Uncle Harry go to the funeral. Joe decides to climb up the apple tree, he collects the apples and cooks them, and he then opens a tin of condensed milk to put over the apples. Both Joe and Dennis are beaten. I am not beaten because I don't like apples and haven't eaten any of them. Joe hates Uncle Harry. I just feel a coldness inside that never goes away.

Joe wants to go home and live with our mother; he keeps running away from the children's home, it does not seem to matter how many times he is punished and brought back, he still keeps running away. The authorities tell my mother that she has to take him back to live with her. Dennis and I can remain in care but Joe has to go. There are a lot of heated discussions about me leaving the children's home, but Uncle Harry and my mother insist that all three of us go home to live with her. I do not want to go. I am about seven years old.

Reflections in Hindsight
On Chapter Two

I now realise just how distressed the children at the children's home were. We had no adults of our own to be attached to and the attention of the members of staff from the children's home became very important. Some children were apparently favoured because they were very young or because they made the staff feel valued. There were also individual preferences, Mummy Robins for instance did not like boys and some children learnt to behave in such a way that the staff felt good about them. It is important to remember that staff would have been untrained, ordinary women and men who were of low status. Perhaps it was a job that was taken up because it provided both accommodation and pay rather than because of any love of children.

For myself, as a result of the psychotherapeutic work that has been done with me over the years, I now can see how devastating was the loss of my little friend, Ruthy, who had enabled me to join in the world of children. Once Ruthy left the Hollies I again became isolated amongst the other children. Mummy Robins was the only person to whom I felt close and who in some sense helped me to feel valued, but also made me an object of envy and hatred with other children.

Under the circumstances my gravitation towards my brothers was inevitable. Touch and comfort would have been important to all of us, however it came about because of the lack of warmth in our environment.
I found out many years later that my brother Joe had already been sexually abused by a member of staff in the children's home, and therefore had a precocious knowledge of sexual behaviour. I am not sure whether Dennis had also been abused.

I find it incredible that the staff were unaware of the physical abuse that was already taking place when my brothers and I went on home visits. We all must have had bruises and marks on our bodies. Corporal punishment was common in those days, but this was at unacceptable level in any time. Perhaps the staff did not want the trouble that it would cause. I think that the culture in the children's home was such that children reporting abuse were considered to be telling lies.

UNHAPPY AT HOME

CHAPTER THREE

No one asked me if I wanted to go with my mother and Uncle Harry, but then I had told them many times that I did not like being with them.
There is a feeling of dread. I am going home. Home, that is where I stay with Mummy Robins, not with my mother and Uncle Harry. My mother's hatred of me is such that she can't bear to touch me. Uncle Harry canes us very hard. I have to watch him and I have to watch what I do because he seems to hit me for no reason, just because he feels like it. It makes my mother cross too and she also hits me, but in the face.
Joe says, "Pamela, you're not to be a baby. You have got to love mum, she is your mum, not anybody else, and mum loves us. Don't muck this up or I'll punch you."
Dennis is excited and seems really pleased that he is going home.
How can Joe and Dennis see my mother so differently, when I can't feel anything about her?
I see her as a very beautiful lady, very pretty. She has dark hair with a red sheen; she is tall and slim and dresses in a way that makes people want to look at her.
The other kids say, "Cor your mum is so pretty."
But she is never there for me. I never see any sign of this love.

I feel numb on the day we leave the Hollies; two big black cars are there to collect us. We are taken to a two bedroom flat on the second floor. It is on a large council estate, called the Woodberry Down estate, at Manor House, London. I feel weird, different from the other kids on the estate. On the first day of school I feel awful. My mother has made me wear a tartan skirt, with a blouse, jumper and clumpy shoes; she also has put a ribbon in my short hair. The other kids all know each other and the term has already started. They laugh at me, I have always been backward and I don't understand any of the work that they are doing. I can't read or write as well as the rest of my class, I am seen as an odd child, withdrawn, stupid and possibly trouble.

The flat we live in is small, sparsely furnished and always cold. All the rooms lead off a small passage; there is a tiny box kitchen, a living room where we also eat our meals, two bedrooms and a bathroom and toilet. The only room that is heated is the front room, which has a coal fire. When we first move into our new home Uncle Harry does not live with us all of the time, on Tuesdays and Thursdays he stays with Nanny Donnelly. I so look forward to Tuesdays and Thursdays. My brothers share one of the bedrooms and my mother and Uncle Harry sleep in the other bedroom. My bed is the put-u-up sofa in the living room. I am put to bed in my mother's bed, early in the evening, and then Uncle Harry carries me into the living room to the sofa bed. I don't have a cupboard or wardrobe for my clothes, although they must be put somewhere.
We are all instructed over and over again, that we are not to tell anyone the family business and especially never to tell anyone that Uncle Harry lives with us.

My mother presents herself as a weak tearful woman. Whenever there is any emotional tension evident within the family she is physically sick with vomiting and diarrhoea. Joe winds her up continually, he sits on top of on the coal cupboard and bangs his feet on the sides of the doors, and my mother pleads with him to stop it.
He laughs at her and says, "Make me, go on you make me".

My mother screams at him and chases him along the balcony and down the stairs. When she doesn't catch him she breaks down and cries. Joe continues to taunt her. My mother tells Uncle Harry about Joe's behaviour and he steps in: a beating with Uncle Jack, a stick that stands in the corner, is a regular occurrence. There is a set time and place, six o'clock, after the evening meal, in the living room. The washing up has been done, and the whole family watches the punishment that is inflicted on whichever child has transgressed. If all three of us are involved, then we watch the other two being beaten until it is our turn. My mother is always expected to be present.

My mother works during the day; Joe is the oldest, so he carries the front door key on a piece of string around his neck. Before we go to school and when we get home from school we all have our jobs around the house to do, washing-up and putting the cups away, making the beds and cleaning the old coal out of the fire grate. Often on the days that Uncle Harry isn't staying at home, the jobs won't get done.
Joe says. "Sod it."
He sets up a boxing ring in the boy's bedroom and I am the referee or we play football in the hallway. It is a rough game, in a small area, grazed knees and bloody noses are frequent but worthwhile.
Sometimes Joe doesn't get home from school until late. I am left sitting on the open stairs that take us up to our second floor flat, I am freezing cold and I dread the consequences of what is going to happen when my mother gets home. My mother often blames me and doesn't hold back from smacking me in the face.
She says, "What are you looking like that for, you're dirty and scruffy. Get out of my sight. I don't want to look at you."

When Uncle Harry returns home she cries and is ill, saying that she can't cope. He then punishes the three of us.

There are always certain foods that we are told are Uncle Harry's.
"You are not to drink the milk, that's Uncle Harry's."
The jam is his, the apples in the fruit bowl are his, the biscuits and many more foods, far too many to list. Sometimes he marks the jam pot or the milk bottle. As soon as the evening meal is finished and my mother and I do the washing up, he lines the three of us up and asks who has touched his jam. We remain silent. He takes out his (John Bull) printing set and takes our fingerprints. He pushes our fingers into the ink and then forces them down, one by one on the writing paper, saying, "If you don't tell me now and I find out it's your fingerprints, it's going to be much worse for you."
Dennis cries, as usual he can't take the tension. Joe often takes the caning even if it isn't him who has eaten the jam, or I say that I have eaten it, if it is me, and it is very often me.

During the school holidays and after school, when the chores are completed and at weekends my brothers are expected to look after me and take me with them wherever they are playing on the estate. There are times when they hate it. They say to me, "You have to keep up with us, run as fast as us, or we will leave you behind, play football like a boy, as well as we play, and you must be able to steal sweets and cigarettes from the shops without getting caught."
I wear Dennis's clothes, his trousers and jumper. He is small for his age and not that much bigger than I am, although he is three years older. I comb my hair back with hair grease so that I look like a boy, and I also act like a boy.

Joe says, "Climb up onto my back, Pam."

He then pushes me through the small window of the fur factory, so that I can open the bigger window and the boys can get in to steal the off-cuts of fur, which they attach to the handlebars of the bikes that Dennis has made up from old dumped bikes. We really do wild things on the bikes, we don't seem to think or care about getting hurt, we weave in and out of the traffic on the main road and catch hold of the back of the Pop lorry, which then pulls us alongside. We are always getting into dangerous things, such as balancing on the main pipe that runs across the reservoir and cycling a long way to play on the train lines.

My brothers push me through the small window of the boys' toilets at the cinema, and I open the side door for them. We are often caught and thrown out.

Mrs O'Shea, a large fat woman who lives in the flat beneath us, frequently complains.

She bangs on the doorknocker and says to my mother, "Those children are out of control."

She tells my mother what she has observed. "And the noise is dreadful; sometimes I think that they are killing each other. The other day I looked through the letter box and there was blood everywhere, they are animals and Joe is the worst of the three."

"Silly cow, fatty O'Shea," I mumble.

The sexual games that we played at the children's home also increase. Joe gets me to masturbate him, and Dennis looks at me naked and touches me and asks me to touch him. The sexual play becomes more aggressive. When we play cowboys and Indians they, the cowboys, capture me, the Indian, take my clothes off, tie me up and masturbate or rub their penises against me. Hitting me with a belt is common, or they tie me to a chair, tell me to keep still and aim darts at my feet to see how close they can get to my

feet without a dart sticking into me. I feel numbness all over my body. It's as if my body does not belong to me.
I am nine years old and I am totally cut off from what is happening. As my brothers throw darts at my feet, when one of the darts sticks into my foot, I don't feel anything.

Dennis starts to invite his friends to join in. I am with Dennis and his friends in the bushes at the back of the block of flats where we live. The boys touch and grab at me. They also put objects like pencils inside my vagina.

I play football with the boys at school. Girls do not play with me, or I have no wish to play with them. In return for being allowed to play football with the boys, at break times I go into the damp dirty pram sheds where I let them touch me sexually. To get to the pram sheds we have to climb through a hole in the school fence and go down into the basement of the flats opposite. The tenants who live in the block of flats are not using many of the sheds and lot of the small pram-shed doors are left open, the boys from school have made little camps out of them, using wooden crates as seats and one wooden crate placed in the middle is used as a small table. On the table is a torch, matches and an oil lamp. It is very dark and there is a musty smell, sometimes it also smells of pee, where one or two of the sheds have been used as a toilet. There are also leaky pipes so the floor is always wet under foot. The torch and the oil lamp make shadows on the wall, which makes my time in the pram sheds very spooky and at the same time exciting.

One of the teachers at school finds out what I have been doing with the boys in the pram shed. My mother is told; the family doctor is called out to my home. I feel stupid and so ashamed, as the doctor looks between my legs. The doctor doesn't speak to me or touch me; he just looks at me and then leaves me in my mother's bedroom, while he goes to talk to my mother in the living room.

Uncle Harry moves into our flat and stays all week, and he also starts to be there during the daytime.
Nanny Donnelly comes to our flat for Sunday dinner; she arrives early enough to help my mother to cook the meal, while Uncle Harry goes to the Manor House pub. He drinks a vast amount of alcohol and still does not appear drunk. The food is put onto the table as soon as Uncle Harry returns home. We wait to see what mood he is in, as to whether dinner is eaten in silence. Joe makes himself scarce, missing dinner altogether. Dennis and I are expected to go to Sunday school as soon as the dishes are washed and put away.
"Go on, piss off and give your mother and me a break, don't come back until after five; I don't want to be bothered by you two or anyone else until then."
Uncle Harry slumps on the sofa to sleep off the effects of his lunchtime drinking.

More often than not Dennis and I don't go to Sunday school where we never feel welcome. This follows an incident where Joe and Dennis had stolen the Sunday collection money. The church, the police and the school were there to join in with the familiar chant of how wicked we all are. "All of you three children have been given chance after chance and people have put themselves out for you. There is your mother who works her fingers to the bone for you and the vicar who tries to help and the staff at the school try to teach you right from wrong."

Instead of attending Sunday school, we wander the streets or if it is raining we play a game of marbles up against the wall of one of the open entrances of a block of flats, or we play a game with cigarette picture cards, which we flick up to a card that is leaning against the wall. The winner is decided by who ever manages to knock the leaning card down. In fine weather a walk down Lordship Road often seems more interesting than staying on the estate. We crouch under the front window of a house and peer through any gap where the curtains don't quite meet, to watch the television. It doesn't seem to matter that we can't hear the programme that happens to be on; we just need to stay out of Uncle Harry's way for a couple of hours. If we are spotted, then it is time to run like hell, we don't want to be caught. That will mean facing Uncle Harry's wrath and that is to be avoided at all costs.

Uncle Harry works as a meat porter. Lumping heavy meat around has developed his physique and, although he is very overweight, he is also a strong muscular man. He is known to his work mates and to his drinking pals in the pub as Tiny. When he enters the pub there is a sense of presence about him. No one ever crosses him or answers him back. I think that he is respected, but perhaps he is feared. Like all bullies he senses fear and exploits the situation. Lots of drinks are bought for him and he is constantly told that he is a great man.

The sexual game playing still continues with Joe and Dennis. Dennis no longer invites other boys to join in, he mostly comes to my bed in the middle of the night and lies on top of me until he has climaxed. Uncle Harry has decided that I am no longer trustworthy and I am not allowed to go out without his approval.

I am seen as odd and backward at school, now I am also seen as bad. The other children's parents tell their children to stay away from both my brothers and myself, the boys because they are bad and always in trouble, and me because I am both mad and bad. At break times I have to stay with the member of staff who is on playground duty and at dinner time I go home where Uncle Harry can make sure that I am not getting into trouble.

Uncle Harry starts work at five in the morning and could be home by midday, unless he goes to the pub after work.

One day when I get home from school, at lunchtime, Uncle Harry has run a bath for me. He says, "Take off your clothes and get into the bath. You are dirty and scruffy and you need to be given a good scrub."

He is right, I always look dirty and scruffy, but I am puzzled because this has never bothered him or my mother before. The bath is hot and steamy and when I get into the bath he washes me, not in the usual rough way that he usually washes me, this time he talks to me in a gentle voice, he takes me into the front room and dries me off with a towel. His eyes look funny, almost glazed with a slight grin on his face. He keeps rubbing my nipples until the pain becomes unbearable.

I brush my chest with my hand, telling him, "It hurts."

His smile broadens and he says, "But you like it, you let the school boys fuck you. You're ready."

He rubbed Vaseline inside my bottom. All I can smell is the baby powder that he sprinkled over my body. He roles me into a ball on the sofa and has anal sex with me. The room goes dark and I see stars, I can't breathe and I think that my neck is going to snap in two, as his heavy weight forces my head into the corner of the sofa.

When he has finished, he tells me to get dressed. His face has changed back, to his normal stern face. I can now smell the cigars on his breath as he cups the back of my neck with his hand and pulls my face close to his.

He says in a snarl, "That's because you let the schoolboys do things to you. You wanted it. You fucking little slag."

He says, as his voice changes into his superior voice, "You must not tell anyone because I will make sure that you are punished and it will kill your mother. You know that she isn't a strong woman and you don't want to be responsible for killing her. Do you?"

There must be a lot of physical pain when he puts his full weight on me and anally abuses me, but I go somewhere else in my head. I am completely cut off.
I feel confused. My head is spinning all afternoon at school. I can still smell his talcum powder that he put on me. My knickers are damp and disgusting.
"He used his talcum powder on me, did this make me special?"
"Smart!"
A voice yells at me. It is Mrs Jennings.
"Where are you girl? Are you in this class this afternoon?"
I look at her blankly. I feel lifeless and distant. Mrs Jennings carries on talking and writing on the board, as her voice drifts in and out of my consciousness.

At home after school, Uncle Harry is in a jolly mood. He puts his arm around my shoulders and pinches the top of my arm.
"Good time at school?" he asks.
"If you pass your eleven-plus I will buy you something special."
I look around at the flat and notice that he has done all the housework, which is normally my job. The vegetables are prepared and sitting in the saucepans waiting to be cooked for the evening meal. He pats the side of my cheek, before starting a play fight with me.
He raises his hands and takes a boxer's stance and says, "Come on, hit me!" as he blocks my small flying fists with his huge hands. This is a game that the boys and I would play.

A while later he looks at the clock on the mantelshelf over the fireplace.

"What's the time?" he asks.

I know that it is about the time that my mother will be coming home from work. I cannot tell the time.

"Six o'clock." My answer came out too quickly.

He laughs and says. "Still can't tell the time then? When you can I will buy you a wristwatch. That will be sometime never." He smirked.

"Do you want to go and meet your mum at the bus stop?"

"Yes!"

I do. This is an unexpected treat.

He says, "You stand at that bus stop.

He points at the Green Line bus stop, which can be seen from the front room window.

"I want to be able to see you. You wait for her to come."

I feel very excited and pleased with myself. I can see my mum walking towards me. I rush up to her and take her shopping bag from her. I feel very special and grown-up.

After tea I go out to play. Uncle Harry says, "You don't have to wash the dishes, your mum can manage. Off you go, play downstairs where I can see you."

He took me to one side. "Never forget. I can always see you. I always know what you are doing and saying. I know everything about you." A shiver runs through me. I believe this big powerful man.

When the ice cream van comes, my mum buys ice cream for us all. This is unusual, I am included.

Uncle Harry having sex with me becomes a regular occurrence. Most weekdays at lunchtime he is there, waiting for me. He forces me to have either anal or oral sex. I vomit and choke, and I hate and dread it. If I co-operate with him he will allow me to go out to play rather than staying indoors to clean the flat or make my brothers' beds or prepare the vegetables for the evening meal.

There are times when I can't face going home from school at lunchtime. My punishment is brutal.

There is a six pm beating after the evening meal, when I have completed clearing the table and have done the washing up for the family. He canes me in the bedroom where my mother and he sleep.

He leaves me in their bedroom after the beating. He says, "You stay here and think about what you have done."

I stand staring out of the window, I can see the flats across the way and I can see two or three girls out playing. They go to the same school as me, and I think that they are so lucky. Sadness wells up inside of me, but I push any tears away. I can't let Uncle Harry see that he can make me cry.

My mother returns to her bedroom after about an hour and tells me to come into the sitting room with her. I don't look at her; it's better for me to look at the floor.

As I walk into the sitting room, Uncle Harry barks at me, "Repeat the seven times tables."

I stutter after "One times seven is..."

He puts his face up against my face until his nose is resting on my cheek and says, "You stupid little bastard. What are you? You're a stupid little cow."

He pulls me by my ear and pushes me to a sitting position in the corner of the room. He forces a pointed cardboard hat that has dunce written on it onto my head and says, "No one is to talk to her, do I make myself clear?"

I sit in the corner wearing the hat all evening and every evening and at the weekend until Uncle Harry decides that the punishment can stop.

Uncle Harry buys sweets and makes a point of handing them around to other members of the family. He lies on the sofa and my mum sits in an armchair to the left of him and Joe and Dennis sit on the floor, in a position where they can see the T.V. Uncle Harry says, "You are wicked, a useless wicked filthy little bitch and you do not deserve to be given treats."

The abusive punishment goes on for days. What hurts me the most is when my brothers join in. As they walk past me, they kick me saying, "Slag, you're nothing but a filthy little slag." My face changes as my bottom lip drops and quivers. My whole face freezes in despondency and despair. Uncle Harry calls for my mother to fetch the camera. He says, "Elsie, get the camera, hurry up and get the fucking camera, we have got to get a picture of this. Stupid little cow."

He holds my chin and forces my face outwards where they can all see me. They all fall about pointing and laughing at me.

There are times when I can't recall where the time has gone. One minute I am sitting here in the corner and the next thing that I know is that it is the next day and I am getting myself ready for school. On other occasions I can see me looking down at myself. I don't feel anything because it's not me. It is someone else sitting there.

At school I am seen as odd and stupid. I only play football with the boys. I can fight as well as any boy in my class. One day I run down the corridor at school and a male teacher whom I don't know but who seems to know me says, "I have been watching you playing football." He turns me over, smacks the tops of my legs and says, "If you want to be seen as a boy, then I will treat you like a boy." I am puzzled; I can't work out the connection! Most of my time at school I spend alone, I am a loner, I sit quietly and am usually away with the fairies, thinking about I don't know what, but I am not on this planet.

My mother begins to look for a secondary school for me. Joe is just leaving secondary school and that school does not want to take me. They say, "We have already had to put up with two members of the Smart family, who are always trouble, and we are not going to put up with a third."

Joe arrived home one day with a bruised, swollen eye and a split fat lip.

"Mr Johnson had a fight with me in the boy's gym. I kicked a cupboard and, as it slammed shut, the cupboard door caught his ear." Joe laughs as he tells me.

"Mr Johnson was so angry that he dragged me by the scruff of the neck over to the boys' gymnasium, fitted me with boxing gloves and told me that he was going to give me the thrashing of my life."

It seems perfectly all right, for a thirty-year-old man to use a fifteen-year-old boy as a punch bag. Joe himself thought that he still scored a point when he trapped Mr Johnson's ear in the cupboard door. I wonder if they would punch me and, after what happened to Joe, I don't want to go there anyway.

My mother disputed the school's decision and the issue was resolved by the Education Department. I am not told the outcome of their decision until the autumn term has started.

Woodberry Down Comprehensive School is a huge grey building. I can almost see it from the balcony where we live. The block of flats opposite to ours hides it. I can see part of the boy's playground and I can see the hundreds of school children who are walking from school towards Manor House tube station.

My first day at Woodberry Down is terrible. All the new children go into a huge assembly hall. As each child's name is called out, they are told which queue to join in. My name is called and I join the line with all the other kids that are in Miss Branch's class. I feel dreadful and my heart is pounding. I don't know any of the other children in my class, there is no one there that I recognise from the junior school or whom I have seen around the area where I live. Miss Branch takes us to our classroom and we are told to find a desk.

When we are all settled Miss Branch says in a loud voice, "Where is Smart, Pamela Smart, where are you?"

I put my hand up. She indicates for me to join her at the front of the classroom. She says in front of the class, "Let's get one thing clear. You are not wanted at this school and I certainly do not want you in my class. I will have you out of my class by Christmas. Sit at the front of the class so that I can keep an eye on you."

I felt so humiliated, stupid and scared. Joe's voice came into my mind:

"Don't cry, don't let these bastards get the better of you. Fight back. Don't be weak. Fight, fight and keep fighting. Do not trust anyone."

I hate Miss Branch, as much as she dislikes me. Any sarcastic or humiliating remarks made by her wash over me without making any impact. In fact I feel more defiant against Miss Branch, my form teacher, than all the other teachers in the classes that I attend. I start to be disruptive in a way that I have never been at junior school.

My disruptive behaviour starts to get me into trouble. I get to school late, turn up dishevelled, wearing no tie, which is part of the school uniform and should be worn at all times, my shoe laces are undone, I haven't bothered to wash and I am generally a mess. When this is pointed out to me I laugh, shrug my shoulders and say, "So what?"

I get to class late, and make a noise by banging doors or my desktop. I cannot be bothered to pay attention in the classroom. My homework is not done. Being caught smoking in the girls toilets and being rude and cheeky to staff are the main offences that the headmistress or my housemaster complains to my mother about.

My mother is called to the school, she looks fragile and frightened. As she cries she says, "I'm on my own and I don't know what to do with her. I do my best for all my children. I can't cope any longer."

She turns to me. "You are making me ill. Do you want me to have a breakdown? You are killing me. I can't take this any more."

I can't look at her for very long because she makes me feel bad. She looks so helpless, like a frightened child. Tears fall down her face and her hands are shaking.

The housemaster says, "I will cane her for you, Mrs Smart, I can see that you need help. She is a very difficult child."

A male teacher does not usually cane girls at school. Sometimes girls are smacked across the back of their legs with a ruler. My mother declines the offer for me to be caned, and I am put on report as usual.

Miss Branch is correct; she does have me out of her class by Christmas. I am put into the remedial class, where I remain for the next eighteen months. This means that I do not go up a year with my peers who are the same age as me. The younger new intake of children joins me in the remedial class.

If I have avoided having sex with Uncle Harry by not going home at lunchtime, I deliberately get into trouble so that I don't have to go straight home after school because I am put in detention, or I will hide behind groups of children, or behind a small wall that runs along the road between the school and the block of flats where I live. I bend down making myself as small as possible and run until I have passed my block of flats where Uncle Harry is standing on the second floor balcony, watching the children coming out of school. I think to myself, "I would rather be beaten than have him groping and touching me in that revolting way. In this way I defer the trouble that is coming."

The worst time for me is games day. I love any sports and I am very good at most sports but after a game of hockey, or track and field events is over we are expected to have a shower. The showers are communal and a member of staff supervises. Sometimes I can get away with not taking a shower by telling the teachers that I have forgotten my towel and wash things. At other times a spare towel and soap is produced for me to use.
The teacher stands there, "Come on, get undressed and take a shower, you manage to avoid taking a shower nearly every week."
I shake my head, defiantly, indicating no.
"You are already on report, Pamela, you know you could be expelled if you don't do as you are told."
I shrug my shoulders. No way am I going to let anyone see these marks on my body, which my clothes hide.
The gym teacher, who I like, marches me to the headmistress's office. The headmistress says to me: "We have doctors' children and children who come from respectable families who attend this school, and I do not want the likes of you in my school."
Her words are wasted. They go right over my head. I stare out of the window.
"Well, what have you got to say for yourself?"
I say nothing.
"You are a waste of my time and if I had my way I wouldn't have you in my school, you are a disgrace. Do you understand? No one wants to waste anymore time on you."
She points at her office door and says in a dismissive tone.
"Go on, get out of my sight. Wait outside my office until I have decided what to do with you."
I wait, dreading that I am going to be forced to take a shower. Not only am I afraid that the teachers or the other

kids are going to see the cane marks on my bottom and back. They will also see how deformed I am. I believe that what Uncle Harry has done to me sexually has deformed my vagina and my breasts. I feel an overwhelming sense of shame.

The punishment that the headmistress decides on is that I can stand outside her office, for a week, instead of having my morning or afternoon break with all the other kids. I got off lightly!

One of my early morning tasks before going to school is to go to one of the newspaper stands to buy the daily newspaper for Uncle Harry. I ran to one of three newspaper stands that are in our area, kicking a ball up against the sidewall as I run along the street. I pick the ball up into my arms and take a newspaper from the stand, I put down a sixpenny piece, then pick up most of the change that is on top of the counter as if I am collecting my change. When I am sent to get other items of shopping for the family, I steal what I can and pocket the shopping money. To my amazement I am never caught.

I also steal from my mother's purse and Uncle Harry's money dish where he leaves all his loose change. I am frequently found guilty of this offence. As a punishment he canes my left hand. As the cane strikes he says, "This is what happens to thieves, if you do this when you get older you will have your fucking hand chopped off."

He canes my left hand so that it will not affect my ability to write or to carry out my household tasks. I can, of course, also continue to touch him sexually.

With the money that I have stolen I buy sweets and cigarettes, or I hide the money inside the lift door, which has a shelf on top of the doorway.

It is the summer holidays and Uncle Harry rewards me for being 'good'. I did what he wanted me to do. I am allowed

out for the day. I tell him some tale about where I am going. "I'm going to Nanny Donnelly's, she wants me to help her unpack some of her boxes."
Nanny Donnelly has moved from Durham Road to Highbury Crescent.

With the stolen money that I have been saving, I buy a Red Rover ticket, which means that I can travel on red London Transport buses to the end of their route. I catch a bus to London Bridge station, and then take the number 9 bus to Sidcup Kent. I feel so excited. I am on my way home to the Hollies and to be with Mummy Robins.
I arrive unannounced. She looks surprised and asks me how I am; she carries on with what she is doing. One of the girls from the house, Cathy, another one of Michael's sisters, asks me what I am doing here, "What do you want? Mummy Robins is my mother now, not yours, so go away."
Mummy Robins seems distant and cold towards me. This rebuff cuts me to the core.
"Where is Michael?" There wasn't any sign of him. "He has been too naughty to stay at Rose cottage. He was moved to another cottage, which has a housefather rather than a housemother." As Cathy tells me, she smiles in triumph.

I leave and go to see Michael. As I walk across the grass, past the cricket pitch and the sand pit, memories of when I was a small child, living at the Hollies, come flooding back. The time when the cricket ball knocked me out, as the bigger boys were playing cricket and I had wandered onto the pitch. When I got locked in the swimming pool because I had decided to hide from Mummy Robbins and she left the pool with all the other kids.

I arrive at Michael's cottage, which is a long walk from Rose cottage. This isn't a part of the Hollies that I know very well. I am invited indoors by an older boy and I see Michael. I hold my breath for a moment as I see him sitting on the floor with his face turned to the wall. I call his name in a whisper and he slowly turns to look at me, he turns towards me with a blank lifeless expression. He does not communicate with me. I don't think that he even recognises me.

I make my way back past Rose cottage and walk up the path towards the main gate. Fragments of memory flicker in and out of my mind.

The woods, with the sunshine dappling through the trees. The trees are my friends and I used to play with them. I pretended that they were my teddy bears and I spoon fed them and talked to them. My safe place, my hideout, which seems just the same as ever, I think to myself. "But why does it make me feel uneasy?" I push the thought away.

As I leave the Hollies I feel deflated.

I walk to a local park. There is a mo-ped with its keys in the ignition. I ride it around the park until I fall off, and then make my way to the bus stop. There is a group of girls from the children's home at the bus stop, they push and punch me until I fall to the ground.

"Thought you would come back and be clever," says one girl.

Another one shouts: "What you looking at? Are you looking at me? Do you think that you are better than me?"

They kick me in the back several times. I don't fight back. It is as if all the fight has been taken from me. I get onto the bus to find that during the scuffle I have lost my ticket.

The conductor asks, "Where's your ticket then, Miss?"

I tell him that I don't have one. "I must have lost it."

"You girls, you're all the same, take me for some sort of fool."

He asks me for my name and address. I give a false name and address. The police take me off the bus and take me home. I must look a mess and I think for a moment that the police have some concern about my welfare.

My mother and Uncle Harry are furious with me when they find out where I have been. The police leave and I say something that my mother doesn't like or look at her the wrong way. She starts to slap and punch me, around my body, and then pulls my hair, so that she can hit me in the face. My mother always wants to hit me in the face when she loses her temper and lashes out. Uncle Harry pushes me and forces me to the ground. As I fall my back slams against the wall with a thud.

The next morning I wake up and I can't move my legs. There is something wrong with my back.

My mother calls for Dennis. She seems to be in a panic. "Dennis," she shouts, "she can't move, she looks limp and unwell. I don't know what to do."

Dennis takes over, he lifts me out of bed and sits me in the armchair, and he tells my mother to phone for the doctor and tells her what to say. My mother calms down, the doctor is called and I am sent to hospital. I am put into a plaster cast from my chest to the bottom of my back.

I remain in a plaster cast for some weeks and my right foot becomes painful to walk on. I start to walk on the side of the sole of my foot, rather than putting my foot flat onto the floor. I feel lifeless. It feels as if I have nothing to live for.

The staff at school and other children look at me strangely, but no one asks me what is wrong with me or makes any contact with me. It's as if they don't want to be involved.

The hospital removes my plaster cast and I receive weekly physiotherapy for some time. The hospital staff begin to suspect that I have a mental problem rather than a physical one.

Despite all of this, sexual abuse with Uncle Harry continues with oral sex or me masturbating him. It makes me feel that every part of me that has been touched by his semen is contaminated and can never be washed clean. This is made worse by the fact that I am more available to him because I am often absent from school. I am away when I have a games morning or P.E. and I take time off to attend hospital appointments.

When I am not attending hospital as an outpatient, or being kept at home by Uncle Harry, I go to school, where I am quiet and withdrawn. I spend most of my time in the classroom gazing out of the window. I don't want to eat or be bothered with anything or anyone. The hospital that I am attending is St. Bartholomew's Hospital. There is some concern shown from the hospital staff about my state of mind.
One of the nurses attempts to coax me out of my silence. I stare out of the window, where I can see Smithfield meat market. This is where Uncle Harry works. The market is empty, work there has finished for the day, but his eerie presence is here with me, he is always with me. I remain silent.
I gaze at the decorative green ironwork on the Victorian front of the building. I picture him at work humping huge dead animals that he drapes over his shoulder. How can I talk about him when he is not only present to me mentally but is there opposite the hospital where he is working?

I am admitted to hospital. The ward that I am admitted to is an adult female ward. The other patients are all much older than me. They look at me and say to each other and to the nurses, "Isn't she a pretty girl? Such a lovely girl, it's a shame that she looks so sad!"
I feel miserable, flat and dead inside. I continue not to eat and, apart from grunts of Yes or No,
I don't have anything to say. I just lie there looking into space. My mother comes to visit, but both my brothers and

Uncle Harry stay away. Instead of my walking improving, I refuse to walk at all.

A psychiatrist starts to come and see me on the ward. I can't hear what he says to me. I don't know that I am even listening to him. He insists that I can walk and that it is all in my mind. He gets me to get out of my bed and slowly walks me up and down the ward. The nursing staff seem cross with me and tell me that I am a time waster. I am sent home.

Life goes back to the way it was before. Because I have lost so much weight, boys show more interest in me and other girls say, "You are so pretty."
I go back to stealing and eating more sweets until I gain weight and my acting out at school becomes worse.
One day a prefect catches me smoking in the girls' toilets with two other girls, Sally and Sandra. We are reported to the headmistress.
"Wait outside my office," she said in an exasperated voice, "I have had enough of you all, I don't want you at my school. I am going to telephone your parents, who can come and collect you from the school and take you home."
We do not wait outside her office, we run away. This is the first time that I have run away from home. One of the girls, Sally, takes us to her home which is also on the Woodbury Down estate, she collects some money and pinches a few cigarettes from a box that has been left open on a table amongst a pile of dirty coffee cups and dirty plates with last night's left over food, that has congealed and stuck to the plates. We then make our way to her sister's ex-boyfriend's home.
We take the tube and when we arrive it is dark and I don't know the area. As I walk through the front door of this big old house, I feel a pang of fear. The house is smelly and dingy and the bare glaring light bulb that shines in the long

passage way shows up the dirty wallpaper in the hallway and it looks even dirtier against the dull brown paintwork.

Sally's male friend rents a room in this big old house. Sally's sister is serving a prison sentence for shoplifting and Sally flirts with Ben. She says, "If Irene finds out, she will kill me but I don't care, I've been having it off with him for months."

Sally was my age, thirteen, and Ben was old, at least twenty-two. The two of them sleep in the double bed whilst Sandra and I sleep on the floor.

The next day, which is a Friday, all three of us are at a loss for what to do, we wander down the street still in our school uniforms, and we sleepily look into the shop windows. Suddenly a police car stops and an officer asks us our names. We are taken to the police station. Uncle Harry with one of my brothers comes to collect me. He says in front of a policewoman, who has been asking me questions about where we had spent the night, "Did you have a good dinner?"

I nodded that I had eaten.

He replies, "Well I have a bloody good afters waiting for you when you get home."

I see the policewoman's face change. She looks at Uncle Harry and then at me. There is a questioning look in her eye. I lower my head in shame.

Uncle Harry looks at the male police officer who enters the room and says, "I would like to donate some money to the police benevolent fund." As we leave he puts some money into a box that is on the counter.

The usual punishment takes place when I get home. My mother says, "I don't know why you are doing this to me, I didn't sleep all night and you make me feel so upset all of the time."

Uncle Harry tells me that I have been suspended from school for six to eight weeks while the school decides what to do with me.

I spend my days cleaning up the house, washing, ironing, cooking and anything else that needs to be done. When the evening meal has been eaten and I have done the clearing up, then I spend the evening sitting in the corner.
I can tune them out; go to some other place in my head. I can see myself sitting there but it is not me.

When Uncle Harry sees fit, he decides that I have spent enough time sitting in the corner, so he tells the rest of the family to leave the room. My mother obediently goes off to potter in the kitchen before going to bed. Dennis goes out and Joe, these days, is very rarely at home.
Uncle Harry talks at me for what seems like hours. It feels as if his face is almost touching mine, I feel his breath on my cheek and I can smell his cigars as I breathe in and out. His eyes bore deep into me. There is a note of righteousness in his voice, as he preaches at me.
"You are bad and evil and I am doing this all for your own good, you have your father's blood inside you and that makes you evil."
His voice goes on and on as he continues talking at me for what seems like hours. I can't hear all the words. His voice is distant and becomes fainter and fainter until I tune him out, so what he says passes straight over my head. I sit there looking down at my hands, which rest in my lap.

The school decides that I can return to school if I go to see a psychiatrist. Uncle Harry talks to me at great length about the dangers of telling the psychiatrist anything about what is happening at home.
"You keep your mouth shut, you don't tell anyone about what happens here. Do you understand? Am I getting this

into your fucking thick head? What happens here is my business, no one else's. These people are all idiots and they aren't interested in looking after the likes of you. I don't want nosy parkers sniffing around here asking questions and upsetting your mother. So shut your gob and remember." His voice changes into a certain chilling tone. "I do know about everything you say or do."

I go to see the same psychiatrist that I had seen when I experienced not being able to walk. I am expected to go to the hospital once a week for one hour. For the first few weeks I sit in silence across the desk from this man. I do the same as I do when sitting in the corner at home. I sit with my head down and say nothing. The hour goes very fast as I go somewhere else in my head, the time just passes, I don't know where I go. When I get home Uncle Harry asks what I have said and what questions the doctor has asked me. I tell him that I didn't say anything. The sexual and physical abuse continues.

On one occasion the doctor suggests that I spend my time drawing. He leaves the room and comes back some time later. I draw a picture of aeroplanes, lots of aeroplanes that are exploding in the sky. Every week I draw the same picture, I start to tell the doctor about the children's home, how when Mummy Robins went on holiday I would wave to all the aeroplanes that passed by in the sky and how I dreaded them crashing and her never coming back. I have been going to see the psychiatrist for about six months when he asks me whether I would like to see a woman doctor. I say that I would.

I don't know why but I feel quite good about seeing a woman doctor and when Uncle Harry asked his usual questions about what I have been talking about with the doctor, I tell him that the next time that I am going to the

hospital, I am going to see a woman doctor. He goes mad. He gets out one of his meat knives, presses the blade up against my cheek and says, "I will cut out your tongue if you tell anyone about anything. Don't you go telling one of those doctors that I live here. You do know that women are worse than men, don't you? They will see you as evil and you will go into care. I will make sure that you don't go back to the Hollies, you will go to where all bad girls go to, it will be like a prison, and it will kill your mother. Can you live with that?"
I shiver with fear; my head goes into a spin as if I have been beaten around my head. I can't believe that I have been so stupid. Why have I told him about seeing a woman doctor?

The following week my headmistress sends for me. I go to go to her office. She says: "I have spoken to your mother, she doesn't think that you need to see a psychiatrist again and I agree with her, time you spend more time on your schoolwork, you don't need to go there anymore."
Any hope that I had of being rescued has been dashed. I know that I am on my own again. Uncle Harry has fixed it, so there is no escape, no way out.

My behaviour at school becomes more vacant and distant. It is as if they have completely given up on me and I have completely given up on this world where I don't belong.
One teacher in particularly starts his class by giving me some money and he says, "Go to the shops and buy me a Mars bar. Have a cigarette or something but do not come back to my class until it has finished. I do not want you here, am I making myself clear?"
I disappear for the morning. I stay around the shops that are next to the school, or I find myself wondering in the green area that is between the school and the reservoir. This place reminds me of the woods at the Hollies,

somewhere that I can hide. It feels like a familiar place. A safe hiding place that is mine. A tune comes into my head, "The teddy bear's picnic". I hum the tune over and over. "If you go down to the woods today be sure of a big surprise". I return to the present with jolt. A feeling of fear engulfs me. My heart is racing as I make my way back to school.

One day another teacher asks all the children in the class what they plan to be doing with themselves when they leave school. One kid, Robert, says, "I am going to work with my father in his carpentry business."
Another says that she is going to work as a nurse. The teacher says, "Smart, what will you be doing when you leave school?"
I shrug my shoulders. Mr Henry says, "What I see for you is that at some point you will land up on Holloway gallows."
The other children in the class laugh. What Mr Henry said freaks me out. He must have noticed and as I leave the classroom he tells me that he is sorry and that he didn't really mean to say what he had said. His words stay with me for many years. That I am so bad that one day I will be hung.

I am very good at sports and instead of going to some classes if a sporting event is coming up I go to the gym to practice. I feel ashamed as my sport's kit is usually smelly where it has been left in the school locker all week, but the sports teacher still picks me for the team. Sports matches take place on a Saturday morning and we meet outside Manor House tube station. If I have 'co-operated' with Uncle Harry I am allowed to go but if I hadn't, then he tells me that I have to go and do the family food shopping, which was my usual Saturday chore.

I hate it when I can't go to the matches, I feel such a fool, so ashamed. I am a tough kid, I don't care about school and rules, I can't let the other kids or the teachers know that this man rules me. I run around the block, miles out of my way so that I won't be seen, but I can't also be longer than it normally takes me to do the first round of shopping. If that happens it gives my mother or Uncle Harry an excuse to slap and punch me around. The first round of shopping is for the early morning bread that has to be bought at a particular baker's shop, in Haringey. The second lot of shopping is the vegetables, potatoes and fruit that are bought at Hicks, the fruit and vegetable shop, at the Nags Head. Then I make my way back to Haringey to buy fish at a specified fish shop for my Uncle Harry's tea. Lastly I am sent to buy anything else that is needed. By this time it is the end of my Saturday.

When I go to school on Monday morning, the sports teacher asks me why I have let her down again. I put my head down, shrug my shoulders and say, "I don't know."
She says, "You have let the sports team down a few times now, and I don't think that you are that keen, so I am dropping you from the team."
This upsets me more than anything else but I don't let it show.
If only she knew how much I enjoyed playing in the school matches... it did matter to me. But I can't tell her I'm trapped. I can't say what is happening at home. Almost as I am thinking that thought, it is pushed away.

There are days when I can't face school. Instead, I spend the morning, sometimes the whole day with Chip, a golden retriever who lives in a basement flat in one of the big houses off Green Lanes, just opposite the doctor's surgery. To collect Chip I knock on the owners' door, to make sure that they are not at home. When they do not reply I climb through the top window. I have to go in head first as this is the only way that I can get through the window. I land on the owner's bed where Chip is waiting. He wags his tail and licks my face all over, I giggle as I let him nuzzle his head under my chin, and it tickles me.

The place is smelly, damp and dirty. I search around for any loose change. I find some, and Chip and I leave by the front door. We stop at the shop and I buy sweets for myself and dog-chocolate drops for Chip from the money that I picked up from his house. We walk to Clapton ponds and Chip runs into the pond for a swim and I join him. I love this dog, I love to cuddle him and I can talk to him at great length.

One day I feel so low, I fetch Chip from his house and take him swimming. I get into the water with Chip and I plan to get out of my depth and drown in the water, or at least, to get very ill. It is a very cold day, not a day for swimming fully clothed. I didn't drown, so I stay in my wet clothes for the remainder of the day and just walk around the park. I don't care about not going home at dinner time. I don't want to be there for Uncle Harry. The school doesn't ask questions about my absences and the usual punishment from Uncle Harry takes place.

I begin to stay away from home more and more. Not just during the day, I now often stay out all night. I either wander the streets until the tube station opens early in the morning, then I can sit on the floor of one of the telephone booths with the door closed, or I manage to sneak down to the platform and ride on the tubes for hours. There are times when I go from carriage to carriage when the tube is inside the tunnel; my hope is that I will fall between the two carriages. The other place where I sometimes spend the night is the piece of wasteland that is between the swing park and the reservoir, the same piece of wasteland that is by the school, just further down from the school.

The night passes so quickly. Sometimes I realize, or the police tell me, that I have been missing for a few days. The

beatings from Uncle Harry have become more violent, he loses control and keeps hitting me until my mother pulls him away. I mumble at him, "Dirty pig, I hate you." My mother punches me, she screams at me, "Shut up. Shut the fuck up."
I wait until I have a clear run at the front door, then I run out of the front door and I am away again.

I have been out all night, my mother finds me in the tube station. She says, "Is it true? Is it true? Tell me, has he been touching you?"
The penny has dropped! I don't know how she has allowed herself to acknowledge what has been going on for years. I don't respond to her question, I just feel dazed.
She says: "Don't worry, I am going to tell him to leave, it will just be you and the boys from now on."
As I walk down the balcony with her I feel terrified. As he opens the front door, he says, "You get inside." He is pointing towards their bedroom where the caning usually takes place. My mother tells him that she has to talk to him, she is wailing and saying, "How could you, how could you do this to me?" It all went quiet. I stare out of the window not knowing what is going to happen. My mother enters the bedroom. He is standing looking sheepishly behind her. She says, "You must not tell, please don't ever tell anyone. I will die without him. I can't live without him." "I promise that I will never tell."

Reflections in Hindsight
On Chapter Three

Writing this account of my life leaves me feeling an overwhelming compassion for my brothers and me, three children who were trapped and showing symptoms of very disturbed behaviour. We had such deep problems, which were unnoticed by the adults who should have seen that we were in terrible danger and they had the power to change our lives. Our cries for help were clear, but remarkably went unnoticed.

Writing down Uncle Harry's words and describing his behaviour towards me has been the most painful thing for me to do. I have needed to acknowledge and face the evil, psychopathic nature of this man. The grip of fear that he held over me throughout my childhood followed me into adulthood. So much so that for most of my life the moment the memory of his words entered my mind I instantly pushed them out, far away from my conscious memory.
I can see how the young me had no option but to disassociate myself and go somewhere else in my mind to escape from the relentless abuse that was inflicted on me by Uncle Harry and my family.

My visit to the children's home took away my last vestige of hope and resulted in an injury to my back, which has always been a problem. I must have been quite obviously depressed over many months, to the point that I went into hospital. Even there, there was no recognition that hospital was better than home for me.

The school, rather than being a refuge and a place of learning for me, compounded the abuse. The teachers labelled me on the basis of the behaviour of my brothers. I was doomed to failure from my first day at secondary school. My response got me into trouble but gave me some power in a situation in which I was otherwise helpless. It is not surprising that I did not show any respect to the teaching staff that treated me with such contempt. It was impossible for me to learn under these circumstances.

It is amazing that the teaching staff did not suspect my home situation, particularly in view of my refusal to have communal showers. Did they never ask themselves why I so adamantly did not wish to reveal my body despite all the sanctions and trouble it brought me? It is strange that the teaching staff did not question my mother's request to stop the psychiatric visits, particularly since there was no sign of any change.

Schools in those days were closed institutions where there was no accountability and they were a law unto themselves. How many other children were labelled uneducable when actually they were in deep distress?

CHAPTER FOUR
ACTING OUT

What he has told me over all these years is right. My mother will die if I tell anyone what Uncle Harry has been doing to me. Joe's voice comes into my mind, "You have to love your mum." At this moment I hate her. I obviously do not matter. I am just the rubbish that she can use to keep Uncle Harry in her life. My brothers don't care, nobody does. Why should I please them? I hate them. Most of all I hate myself.

My world goes mad, no more beatings, no more sex with Uncle Harry or the boys. It all stops. They don't have any control over me. I run away from home all the time and when I run away I do not stay in the local area. I hitchhike all over the country. The men who give me lifts are paid by me having sex with them. I travel to Leeds, Birmingham, Manchester and many more places. The police pick me up and return me home. I laugh at the police and at my mother. I goad her and say to her: "Well, you got what you wanted. I am having sex all over the place."

I taunt her and tell her what the men looked like. One time I show her a photograph of two Chinese sailors that I have spent the week with. She looks at me but says nothing. She is powerless to do anything.

I hitch a lift to Liverpool. I love Liverpool, the Beatles, Cilla Black and all the other Liverpudlian musicians. Their songs play in my mind. The words of their music have meaning for me. It touches on how I feel. "All my loving, I will send to you. All my loving, darling, I'll be true." These words are a message for my mum.

This is the place to be. I get to know one or two other young people who are also sleeping rough. They come from the area and seem to look after me. They take me to a housing estate where there are derelict houses, we sleep there at night. It's bleak and cold. Sam, one of the kids, makes a bonfire in the middle of one of the rooms in the derelict house and I curl up on the cold damp dirty floor. During the day I spend most of my time with the other runaways around the dock area. My plan is to get a boat over to Ireland, but for now I go back and forth on the ferry that crosses the Mersey.

On one of the trips on the ferry an old lady who I have been talking to leaves her purse in the ladies toilets. I pick it up. As I get off the ferry I am stopped by the police. They also stop the other girl I am with. The police put us in the back of the police car and drive us to the police station. I stuff the stolen purse down the back of the seat in the police car.

Once inside the police station we are questioned. Where do I live, how old am I and what am I doing in Liverpool? I give them a false name and a lot of nonsense answers. The lies trip off my tongue with ease. A policewoman produces the purse that I stuffed down the back of the seat. She asks me, "Do you think that you are clever?"

I am charged with theft and I have to give them my correct name. I am fourteen years old, too young to be remanded in a police cell, so I am taken with the other girl to a remand centre. When we get there we are told to wait inside a room whilst the police speak to the member of staff. I try the door that leads to the garden. It is open, so we run and run until we get far away from that place. I can't be very bright because the next morning I go back to the ferry port. The police are waiting there and I am re-arrested. The police tell me that I am also going to be charged with breaking and entering. I can't work out how I can be charged with this offence as nothing has been broken and I left the building through an open door.

My mother and Dennis travel up to Liverpool and are there when I appear in court. I am called into the courtroom. It's so formal. There are lots of seats, but most of them are empty. I sit in this box that is higher than all the other empty chairs and higher than where my mother and Dennis are sitting. This man tells me to stand up and the judge walks in and sits at his bench, which is opposite me. I can't stop laughing. There isn't anything to laugh about, but I laugh out loud. The judge is furious and says: "This isn't a laughing matter young lady!" I laugh even more. I laugh so much that I miss what is said.

I am on a train with my mother and brother. My mother tells me that the judge has ordered me to attend a juvenile court in London. I tell my mother that I need the toilet. My plan is to get off the train and run. Dennis follows me to the toilet and without any warning he grabs the back of my hair and drags me back to my seat. Still holding onto my hair he says, "If you upset mum any more I will punch your face in."

I can't remember returning home, I must be completely out of it and I have lost time. I find myself at Cumberlow Lodge, a remand centre for girls under the age of sixteen. Cumberlow Lodge is a secure unit; all the doors on the outside of the building and some of the doors inside are locked. The unit is divided into sections. Two main members of staff run the section where I am placed. There is a communal living room, small dormitories, bathrooms and toilets. Each girl is given a set of clothes to wear. It is like wearing a school uniform. Every morning we are given certain areas to clean and from Monday to Friday we go to school, which is in a different part of the building. There are also craft classes in the evenings for those who want to attend.

Once I have gone through all the formalities and settled in at Cumberlow Lodge, I begin to realise how rough it is. Some of the girls are really tough. They curse and swear at anyone who gets in their way. I carelessly walk across the corridor and step over a section of the floor that had just been cleaned. A scrubbing brush followed by a bucket fly past me, narrowly missing my head. A voice with an Irish accent screeches at me, "You stupid fucking eejet, I have just cleaned this floor. Now fuck off out of the way." I soon learn to keep my distance from Joan and her pals.

A fight breaks out and to my surprise a lot of staff appear and the girls who are fighting are separated. One of the girls continues to shout and scream at the other girl: "I'll get you, you wait, you fucking bitch." She is warned to calm down. Her anger turns onto the staff that are holding her back from hitting the other girl. "Let me go. You just let me fucking go." She kicks out at them, her legs seem to go everywhere and her kicks make contact with one or two members of staff. They bundle her into a padded cell.

This girl is in the same class as me and when I see her a few days later she starts to talk to a group of us during the break. She tells us that her name is Jean and goes on to tell us how she has landed up at Cumberlow lodge. We all listen keenly, wanting to know what she has to say. Jean says, "My mum and dad were killed in a car crash a few years ago, so I went to live with my older sister and her husband, but he started to touch me up. He then started to come into my bedroom when my sister was out at work in the evenings. I told him to leave me alone and I told my sister what he was doing, but she didn't believe me. I ran away and slept rough until this man let me move in with him. I was in the pub with him one night when the landlord phoned the police and the police brought me here."

Other girls also speak about how they had landed up in a remand home. Fights at home, parents who didn't care about them and others who were being abused. I keep quiet.

There is a games morning and as we file out of the door in a single line there is a line of staff blocking the way of any possible runners. The sports ground is like a large asphalt tennis court without the tennis net. To be able to escape, firstly the girl who is running would have to get past the line of staff and then climb a high gate.

I only experience an escape once at Cumberlow Lodge and I am involved. It happens by chance. A group of girls, including me, go to the teaching block for a lesson. The visiting tutor is rather elderly and very gentle, so pupils tend to take advantage of her. Mrs Green enters the room by an external door as we come into the classroom by the internal door, both arriving at the same time. Two of the really tough girls, Joan being one of them, push Mrs Green out of the way, shouting for others to follow them. There is an open door and I run out of it before the member of staff who is accompanying us to the class can reach me and secure the door. I climb over the gate and run as fast as I can. I don't know the area and it isn't long before a police car stops in front of me and I am wrestled to the ground and returned to Cumberlow Lodge. The superintendent is furious with me. I am punished by a loss of privileges: I can't watch T.V. in the evenings and can't attend any evening craft classes. I guess he is also upset because Joan and another of the girls do get away and are not caught for many months. Whilst I am at Cumberlow Lodge reports are written about me and an assessment is made of the most appropriate placement for me.

I am sent to a children's home in South London and put on probation. As soon as I arrive I am off again, living rough in the West End of London. I play dangerous mind games with myself. I see a lorry that has stopped at the traffic lights. I think: can I crawl underneath it and reach the other side before the lights change to green and the lorry will start up again? I throw myself in front of cars to see what will happen to me. I usually bounce off the car with just bruising, and in my mind I go back to Woodberry Down School and see myself floating off the roof. "That will teach them all," I think to myself.

A group of men picks me up with another runaway girl, they give us drugs, and there are hazy bits that I can only half recall of different men taking turns in having sex with me, some sort of gang rape, putting things inside me and oral sex. The other girl and I are blindfolded and taken from the house where the rape takes place. We are dumped by the roadside. Hours have passed before the police pick us up from the doorway in which we are slumped.

I am sent back to Cumberlow Lodge and the doctor there talks to me about the dangers of sexual intercourse.

Whilst I am at Cumberlow Lodge this time, part of their assessment is to see whether I will try to run away again. I am asked to clean the main entrance of the building, where the front door is continually being opened to let people in and out. I know that I am being watched and I make no attempt to run away.

I am returned to the Juvenile Court where I am placed on a hospital order. "What is a hospital order?" I ask.

"Wait in there," says one of the policewomen who are looking after all the girls who have been returned to court from Cumberlow Lodge. I wait in the same room which I waited in before going into the courtroom. I know the drill. All girls will wait here until we have all been into court.

Jean bursts though the courtroom door shouting, "You fucking bastards. No, no, you can't send me to an approved school. I have done nothing wrong. It was him, why are you punishing me? It's not fair. It's just not fucking fair." Jean's shouts have turned into sobs. A woman who must be a court official leans over and says to Jean: "Now, now, it's not that bad. You are going to an approved school for your own protection."

I arrive at a huge bleak building in the back of a police car. I am puzzled when the police car stops and the door is opened by a woman in a nurse's uniform. She says, "Hello Pamela, we have been expecting you. You come along inside with me, we are going to be taking care of you for the next few months."

I follow her through a large door and walk behind her up a flight of stairs. My instinct is to run but the two policewomen who are close behind me block my exit. The nurse presses the bell that is situated on a door on the first landing. The sign on the door reads 'Caesar Ward'. I can hear a lot of keys jingling as the door is unlocked. The nurse pushes the door open and waits for me to follow her. Panic engulfs me. I shout out, "You are fucking joking if you think that I am staying here." My arms and legs kick out as I scramble to get away. I am aware of lots of people holding me on the ground. My clothes are removed with speed as an injection is plunged into the top of my bottom.

I wake up to find myself lying on a bed in a large ward. It takes me a while before I can focus my eyes. I feel slightly blurred and as I attempt to get off of the bed my head spins. The same nurse who met me at the police car says, "You're awake, are you? Now take it easy because you might feel giddy for a while. We had to give you something to calm you down. That's what happens here when you make fuss. Now just you remember that, won't you?"

In time I discover that the psychiatric hospital that I am in is in South London. The ward that I am on is a locked ward, and there isn't anyone else here that is my age. The other patients are old, at least twenty-five and over. They all seem very odd. One woman paces up and down the ward, while another sits mumbling to herself. As I scan the ward I can see a seating area, a dining room area and two rows of beds down one end of the ward. Each patient sits as an individual not communicating with anyone else. I manage to get myself to the toilet and back to my bed.

The next morning I am called into a room where there are lots of strange people sitting down. The doctor, who seems to be discussing me, doesn't talk to me on a one-to-one level. He talks about me and what treatment they are going to give me. Not one of them speaks or looks directly at me, except when I am told that I can leave the room. "Thank you, Pamela, you can leave now," says the ward sister.

Over the next few weeks I am given large doses of Largactyl and I remain on the locked ward. I remain quiet, watch what is going on around me and gaze out of the window. I rarely speak to anyone and apart from the nursing staff no one attempts to talk to me. My mother visits me on Saturday afternoons, and I sit in silence with her.

I manage to steal cigarettes butts from the ashtray used by both staff and patients. I feel so numb, apart from a crying pain deep inside my tummy. As I sit here, I burn myself with a lighted cigarette butt. I burn a love heart shape into my skin. I don't feel any pain as my arm starts to blister. I mumble to myself over and over how much I love my mum and my brother Joe. The sister of the ward appears. She says, "Now stop that at once." The crying pain in my tummy builds up into a huge rage. I feel I have an amazing amount of strength that is bursting through. I start to smash everything that I can come into contact with. Cups that are on the table are swept away with one sweep of my arm. I pick up chairs and hurl them down to the other end of the ward, tables are tossed on their sides and my fists pound against the walls. I make a run towards the windows and smash the windows by punching my fist through them. Nurses who have appeared from nowhere pull me to the ground and give me an injection. I am put into a padded cell.

I remain in the padded cell for a couple of days. The ward sister unlocks the cell door and says, "Are you ready to come out? Can you behave yourself?"

I am returned to the locked ward. I soon learn that there are ways of getting out of this prison. If I am quiet and well behaved, then the staff let me out. There are times that I find myself pushing my way through the door as it is being unlocked for another patient or for a member of staff. When I push my way out I have to run as fast as I can. I run with speed down the stairs and out through the main gate before the man who lets people through the main gate is warned to stop me. I turn and laugh at those idiot nurses who are trying to prevent me from leaving. I do not know why but I always remain in the same area. I never take off around the country as I have done in the past when I ran away from home. I return to the hospital under my own steam or I am taken back by the police.

When I return I tell the staff, or particularly my mother, what I have been up to during the hours or days that I have been missing. I take delight in telling the staff and my mother about acts of self destruction: getting very drunk with men who bought me drinks in return for sex, or injuring myself. I say with a grin on my face, "Look, I've cut myself again." Or I show them the bumps and bruises on my arms. I tell them how I threw myself off of moving buses. I describe to my mother in detail about a sleazy nightclub in the Soho area. I laugh in her face as I say, "I managed to get into the nightclub and no one bothered to ask me any question. There were all these men there and guess what they wanted?" I shout out loud so every one can hear me, "Yes, you guessed right, they were doing it all over the place. But that's what you want, isn't it? You want me to fuck all the time, don't you?" My mother runs out of the hospital crying and I laugh and laugh at her.

As well as getting high and self-destructive there are times when I feel very low. I never cry. It is as if I have never learnt how to cry. I just become very morose and sullen. I listen to sad music on the radio, love songs and think about my mother. The words in the songs go over and over in my head. "Anyone who had a heart would love me like I love you and would be true, true." Or the Beatles song: "Love, love me do, you know I love you, so please, please do, love me do. Ow ow love me do". I shout out to the world: "I love her. I love my mum." My head goes into a complete frenzy and I smash it against the wall, over and over again. My sadness has turned to rage and I am completely out of control.

These outbursts can happen inside the hospital or outside in the street. If they happen inside the hospital, lots of staff appear, I am forced to the ground and given an injection, then placed in a padded cell until I calm down. When the nursing staff are particularly fed up with me I remain in the padded cell for a couple of days. As they open the door they say, "Are you going to behave yourself? If you are, you can come out". There are times when I go into rages outside the hospital. The police arrive and I am either taken to the police station or back to Cumberlow Lodge, then returned to the hospital, or sent straight back to the hospital.

They give me E.C.T. I don't know what that is and I don't know what to expect. I am not aware of what's going on. I am given an injection into a vein in my hand and I go to sleep. When I wake up I can't lift my head up. I am given a glass of water, which I drop. I find it difficult to stand and I walk around in a complete daze for days. My speech is slurred. It is as if I have been hit over the head with a hammer. I begin to dread the thought of them doing this to me again. I am given E.C.T. again and as the day approaches I tell the nurses how much I hate it. I plead with them and when that fails I fight with them. I swear at them and attempt to kick and punch them. "Piss off, leave me alone. I hate this place and I hate all of you." But there are too many of them to fight off and I am strapped down onto a bed and given an injection into my arm. I think that this happened to me five or six times in all.

I meet a male nurse whilst I am strolling in the grounds. I have seen him before, but I can't remember where. I know that he works at the hospital, but not on the same ward that I am on. He asks me if I can meet him outside the hospital. I do and he takes me to a house where there are some other men. He gives me a large glass of vodka and asks me if I want some drugs. He says, "Do you want to try some of these pills? They will help you to feel relaxed." I agree to try some. I will take anything so that I can be off my head. Then I don't have to be me. I hate me! The next few days are a bit hazy, I remember the men touching me and having sex with me although it's all a bit blurred. I can't recall how I make my way back to the hospital. It's now three or four days later and I still feel woozy as if I am still drugged.

When my mother comes to visit me at the hospital, I do what I normally do. I goad her and tell her about what I can remember of the time that I spent with the male nurse and his friends. My mother says, "You are disgusting. I don't want to listen to you any more. You make me ill. Do you understand how awful you are?"

"I don't care what you think of me," I screech at her, "I hate you, I hate everyone." Nurses appear and I am given another injection.

The next thing that I recall is being very sleepy. I have been moved to another ward. I am naked and one of the nurses is washing me while a patient from the ward is changing my bed. I have wet the bed. I don't understand what is going on. I feel all floppy and I can't speak. The nurse who is washing me gets me into a clean nightie. Then she spoon-feeds me and puts me back to bed. She tells me that I am having sleep therapy.

I am conscious again. My mother has come to visit me. I am sitting up in a chair behind a table. My mother is sitting next to me. As I start to come around from this drug-induced sleep, I find it difficult to focus and hold my body up straight, and as I look at my mother I become conscious that she is crying. She says through her tears, "I am sorry. I am so sorry." I am taken aback. I think for a moment: Is she, is she saying that she is sorry for Uncle Harry abusing me or choosing him over myself? She continues, "I am so sorry that I tried to kill you, this is what all this is about. When I was pregnant with you I tried to kill you. Your father thought that you were not his child. He said that I had been unfaithful, so I had to get rid of you. I threw myself down the stairs in an attempt to kill you. I put knitting needles up inside myself and took very hot baths and drank gin in an attempt to get rid of you."

I couldn't believe what she was saying. Everything seemed to be happening in slow motion as if my brain was refusing to hear her words. With an enormous amount of energy I raised from my drug-induced stupor and with a huge feeling of rage I lifted the table and tossed it across the room and shouted, "No. No." The nursing staff dragged me back to my cell as my mother was told to leave. The sister said, "What did you say to her? Go on, please leave, leave now."

The next time that I regain consciousness I am told by a nursing sister who I have not met before, "You are going to court this morning. I'm the nurse who is going with you so I don't want any trouble."
I don't feel as sleepy as I have done over the past few weeks, I can walk unassisted and I think to myself, "Have they reduced the amount of drugs that they are giving me?"
A car arrives and the nursing sister and I get into the car. I stay silent as the nursing sister tells me that I am being taken back to court. She explains, "The doctor doesn't think that this hospital is the right place for you and the court will decide what is going to happen to you."
I am taken straight into the courtroom to the magistrate, no waiting in the waiting room with all the other girls at the juvenile court. Once in court I hear the psychiatrist who has been in charge of my treatment telling the magistrate that I am a danger to myself and a danger to others and in his opinion I should be sent to a special hospital. The magistrate is very cross and says, "I think that it is most inappropriate to send a young girl of this age to a special hospital." The psychiatrist, who is a little man in height as well as in build, looks even smaller.
I am told to leave the courtroom. I leave telling anyone who is listening that I love my mum and my brother Joe. I repeat it over and over again. I am called back to the courtroom. I am told that I am going home for a period of time and that I will be returning to court at a later date.

When I return home my mother tells me how upset she was about being told to leave the hospital and how she cried all the way home. I no sooner return home and walk into their bedroom, the punishment room, when I take a massive overdose of largactyl. My mother tries to make me sick by forcing me to drink salt water. I spit it back into her face. I am taken to a local hospital by ambulance. I must have been unconscious for some days. The hospital staff are very angry with me, as is the magistrate from the juvenile court when I am taken there straight from hospital. I am remanded and sent back to Cumberlow Lodge.

When I arrive at Cumberlow Lodge this time, instead of joining the other girls in the usual section where I had been held before, they take me through many locked doors to a part of the building that I had never realised existed. I am put into a small room that just has a bed. There is a small window through which I can just about see some trees and sky. A member of staff comes and supervises me taking a bath. She says in an Irish accent, "Do you know, Pamela, you are amazing, not like some of the other girls who come here. Every time you come in here you are always so clean, your underwear is clean and all your clothes look as if they are brand new." I think to myself, "Yes, I can't stand being dirty and I have been stealing clothes for years. Every time I ran away and all the time that I was in the psychiatric hospital I stole underwear and clothes to wear so that I didn't have to feel unclean. When on the run, I managed to find places to wash or take a bath." But I was not about to tell her anything.

I am taken back to my room and left until a member of staff brings me dinner with liquid medication that I have to take. After they have locked me in my room, I hear a lot of voices coming from the room next door. A girl is screaming and swearing at the staff telling them to go away. After a lot of noise and banging around, with the girl screaming at them, it all goes quiet. At four o'clock my room is unlocked and I am taken downstairs to a sitting room for an hour. The same Irish member of staff tells me that this will be the routine during my stay here. She tells me that there are other girls in this section of Cumberlow Lodge. This is the secure wing and they are afraid that I am going to harm myself. Therefore I am going to be kept in this wing so that they can protect me from myself. I am warned that if I misbehave I will be put into a padded cell like the girl who is in the room next to me.

A week has passed and I am still on the secure wing at Cumberlow Lodge. Mrs Edwards comes to see me in my room. She says, "What have you been up to now?" I like Mrs Edwards, who is a strict but fair woman and who seems to like me.

She comes back to my room later in the day with some magazines. She tells me that she has been on leave for a week. She talks to me about her sons who are still at school but have Saturday jobs. Mrs Edwards comes and takes me out for a walk around the grounds. She links her arm through mine. She is a tall strong woman and she holds on to me tightly, so there is no chance of me running. I tell her how boring it is being locked in a room for most of the day with just magazines to flick through but she says, "It is for your own good and the staff have to make sure that you are safe."

When I leave Cumberlow Lodge Mrs Edwards comes to see me. She says, "You're a good kid, Pam, not like some of the girls we get in here. You must be good because you are coming up for sixteen and you probably won't be sent back here if you get into trouble again. You might be sent to borstal or prison."

I leave Cumberlow Lodge and I arrive at another psychiatric hospital in South London. Not long after I arrive here, I overdose again with some epilepsy tablets that I have bought over the counter at the chemist in the high street. I have had my stomach washed out and I am to stay in the hospital under observation. My probation officer, Mrs Philpot, comes to visit me at the general hospital. Mrs Philpot is visiting me more often these days. She frequently came to see me at Cumberlow Lodge although I did see her a few times whilst I was in the other psychiatric hospital. She seems to come and go without having much of an impact on me. On this occasion Mrs Philpot sits by my bed and says, "What do you think you are doing young lady? Do you understand that if you mess this up, if you get thrown out of this hospital you can land up in prison or somewhere worse?" The statement that the schoolteacher had made to me at secondary school comes back to me. "Smart, you will end up on Holloway gallows."

I am returned to the psychiatric hospital. The staff here are very cold towards me. I thought the other hospital was bad, but this is scary. I feel distanced from other people, especially the nurses and doctors. They tell me that I am going to have another course of E.C.T. This time I don't fight them. Just before the needle is going to be put into my arm a panicky feeling takes me over and I say, "Please make sure that I am asleep before you put that thing on my head," pointing to the trolley of equipment they have covered with a cloth. The doctor replies, "You should try behaving yourself, then we would not be doing this." I am given the E.C.T. and I am convinced that they don't ensure that I am completely unconscious. I have recurring nightmares and fragments of memories of shaking violently and that my head is hurting me like mad. I become very compliant, almost like a robot. The days just drift by. When

I am told that I am going to be given E.C.T. I just accept the fact that this is what is going to happen today.

REFLECTIONS IN HINDSIGHT
On chapter four

My mother's refusal to get rid of Uncle Harry was a powerful rejection of me and her actions made it seem as if all that he had done to me over the years and all that I had suffered meant nothing.

I think at that time I began to have a breakdown and acted out all my anger and distress. The relaxation of all controls meant that there was no longer the terrible fear of Uncle Harry's revenge. I was never conscious of the anger and it is only while writing this that I see how very angry was the behaviour that I exhibited at that time although I was not aware of it. I also was clearly seeking revenge against my mother, for her utter rejection of me.

I can see it now as an anger rooted in pain and distress. The anger that I actually felt was towards myself and it resulted in a rampage of self-destructive behaviour. Not only did my mother think that I was worthless, so did I. The result was that I didn't care what happened to me to the extent that I continuously put myself in dangerous situations.

It was standard practice in the early nineteen sixties to send girls to approved schools because they were seen to be in moral danger. Frequently accusations of sexual abuse were not taken to be true.

In the psychiatric hospitals I was frequently given E.C.T. against my will and it was used as a punishment. These psychiatric hospitals were closed institutions and both in my case and often-recorded cases various types of abuse were rife and there were no outside controls. The word of a member of staff was always taken over that of a patient.

The male nurse who abused me kept his position of trust, kept his job and I, a fifteen-year-old adolescent, was to be punished and kept quiet by being sent to a Special Hospital for the criminally insane. Had I actually been sent there I might never have been released for many years. I am often grateful for the wisdom and understanding of the magistrate who so strongly opposed the opinion of the psychiatrist.

After I was finally released from any hospital treatment, my spirit had been broken and I responded to life with an unfeeling and unthinking compliance.

CHAPTER FIVE
A FAMILY OF MY OWN

There is no hope of making anyone see how awful life is for me. My mother and Uncle Harry behave as if nothing that has happened to me is anything to do with them. It is surreal. Their life hasn't changed. I think maybe it's me, maybe it was all in my mind. But I know that it wasn't. I mustn't think about it anymore. I've got to be good. I hate it here. I must get away.

Six months have passed and I am back home, living with my mother and Uncle Harry. I am surprised to learn that Joe has got a girl pregnant. He has married her and his wife and son are also living in this small flat with us. Gail, Joe's wife, and their son sleep in the front room with me. The front room is supposed to be my sleeping space but as usual I'm never asked if it's all right by me, I'm just told that this is what is happening until Joe, his wife and son are allocated a council flat. I hate being back here and I know that I have to get out. Maybe Joe has the right answer. If I find a boyfriend and have a baby, I can also get a place of my own. That would be a perfect solution.

My mother and Uncle Harry help me to find a job, nothing that is too taxing, a junior in an office, just a small firm off Hornsey Road. I open the mail, go and get the sandwiches from the hole in the wall café at break time, make the tea and frank all the mail before it goes out in the evenings.

It takes me some time before I feel confident enough to go out with other people of my own age. Kim, a girl that lives on the same estate, invites me to go to the cinema with her. I don't know Kim very well although she went to the same school as I did and at some point I was in the same class as her, even though she is a year younger than I am. Kim lives on the tenth floor of a high-rise block. The lift is often out of order and I find it a struggle to climb the ten flights of stairs. I feel that I have much less energy now. Before going into the psychiatric hospital I would have sprinted up the stairs two at a time, but now I feel lethargic. I don't argue or get angry neither do I get overly excited about anything. I just feel flat.

Kim is an only child and her parents, who are in their late fifties, allow Kim to have friends around. They trust her and they believe her when she spins them a tale about where she has been or where she is going and whom she is going with. When I am at Kim's house I meet up with other friends of hers and one or two boys in a group rather than just the two of us.

Uncle Harry makes no attempt to touch me although he is still crude and still makes inappropriate sexual remarks to me. When George, a boy that I have met through Kim, comes to call for me one evening Uncle Harry beckons me into the kitchen. "Come here. I want you," he says.
George remains waiting for me outside on the balcony. Uncle Harry takes out one of his meat knives, moves close to my ear and says in a whisper, so my mother and George won't hear, "See this?" pointing to one of the knives. "I will chop his dick off if he comes anywhere near you." He picked up a long bladed knife and waved it in my face saying, "I will twist this up inside you if you let any of them touch you." He doesn't shock me. I don't even feel angry. I push his words out of my mind and withdraw inside myself as I did when I was a child. My friendship with both Kim and George fizzles out. I think they find me boring.

One of Kim's friends, Mary, goes around with a crowd of teenagers who are into rock and roll music and although I am invited by Mary to join in with this crowd of young people, I feel out of place. I'm not that interested in rock music and I never have much to say for myself. I can't dance and I feel like the ugly duckling in this crowd.

It's Saturday evening and I'm at a dance. The rock group is playing very loud music and it's so dark in the dance hall I can hardly see the person standing next to me although I am aware that the same lad has been standing next to me for most of the evening. A group of us all leave the dance hall at the same time and get on a bus heading towards Finsbury Park. The lad, who has been standing next to me, sits next to me on the bus. He tells me that his name is Simon and asks if he can see me home.

Simon is a little taller than my five foot four inches. He has amazingly beautiful blue eyes with thick dark eyelashes, which redeem an otherwise unremarkable face. He tries to dress like a rocker in jeans and leather jacket but somehow it never quite comes off. Even in his working suit he always looks awkward. Indeed he is awkward in his actions. He isn't part of the crowd. With the exception of two friends that he went to school with, the other lads tend to ignore him. Simon is a fish out of water, but so am I and that's what drew us together.

He is different from other lads that I have met and I never feel threatened by him. Simon seems such a clever young man to me. He has three O levels and he works in an office, unlike most of the other boys that I know, who work with motorbikes or cars or in factories. Simon lives off Fonthill Road, a road that leads onto the council estate, where he lives with his mum, dad and James, his younger brother. Simon tells me that his father is a builder and wants Simon to become an architect. Simon just wants to be like all the boys that he knows, even though he doesn't fit in.

My brothers see Simon as a bit of a weirdo and Uncle Harry makes fun of him and thinks he is a joke. Simon can't be any sort of threat to Uncle Harry, but still Uncle Harry has to spread his foul poison. He says, "What do you see in him? He isn't a man. He's a weakling. You could have at least found yourself a proper man who enjoys football and can look after himself. I would only have to blow on him and he would fall over. What a fucking joke." He laughs to himself.

Simon takes me home to meet his parents. They don't hide their hostility towards me. They tell Simon, in front of me, that they are disappointed with Simon for getting involved with a girl like me. They ask, "Who is she? Where has she come from? She is a girl with no history!" When Simon's father finds out that Harry Donnelly is my stepfather and my real father is Billy Smart he is even less impressed by the fact that his son is going out with me.

The criticism from Simon's parents manages to shake my already fragile view of myself. It hurts me, whereas my mother's dislike and indifference towards me and Uncle Harry's vile persecution of me fall on deaf ears. Simon has encountered his father's disapproval before and it only makes him more determined to go against his parents. He argues with them, he tells them, "This is my life and I will go out with who ever I choose to go out with." Simon and I continue to see each other every day after work and at weekends and we start to make plans about how we can live together, and actively try to make a baby together.

I have a new probation officer now that I have moved from South London back to my mother's flat in North London. She is gentler than Mrs Philpot. She talks to me and takes her time to listen to me, rather than telling me what I should do or think. When I tell her about my dreams and aspirations of starting a family with Simon she warns me not to get my hopes up, but my hopes are raised and I am convinced that this is my only path to freedom and happiness.

She visits my mother and me at home and as she stands chatting to my mother in the small kitchen. I hear her say, "I am amazed in the transformation of Pamela, she isn't acting out any longer and she is so placid and compliant. The hospital treatment seems to have worked for her." She turns and smiles at me. I don't respond. I don't have anything to say to her or my mother.

Within eighteen months of leaving the psychiatric hospital I am going to marry and I am expecting my first child. Simon's mother and father's opinion of me has not changed. They call me every derogatory name that they can think of. I am a slag, a slut, rubbish, a piece of filth and certainly not the girl that Simon should marry. Simon's father says to Simon in front of me, "Are you sure the baby is yours? It could be anyone's, you know. How do you know that she isn't trapping you?"

Surprisingly there is no reaction from my mother and Uncle Harry, except that Simon must marry me. I think my mother is glad to get rid of me.

Simon and I are married at Stoke Newington registry office on the 30th of December 1967. We move into two rooms on the first floor of a big old house in Hackney. I carry on working as an office junior, my probation order is lifted and we make our new home as comfortable as we can afford.

Jay, my son, is born on the 5th of July 1968. Both Simon and I are now eighteen years old. As Simon arrives home from work, I tell him that I think that the baby is coming. Simon phones for the ambulance and we are taken to the Mothers' Hospital, in Clapton. Simon waits with me in the delivery room until one of the nurses asks him to leave. It is a long delivery, over twenty-four hours, and when my son is born I am exhausted, as is my baby. Baby Jay has problems with his breathing and the nurse rushes him off to the other end of the delivery room. I am so alarmed that I almost jump off the delivery table in panic. The nurse who is still with me looks worried and I think she thinks that I am going to freak out. She says, "It's O.K., Pamela, the baby has had a long journey and he just needs some oxygen to help him to breath." She manages to calm me down.

The doctor arrives to insert stitches inside me, where I have been torn. Whilst giving birth, he tells me that baby Jay's attack was either to do with the long delivery or that Jay might have inherited asthma from Simon, who has a mild form of asthma.

I am soon holding my son for the first time. He looks like a little old man, he has a mop of dark hair and extra long dark eyelashes. He has the look of Simon's dad, only baby Jay is more wrinkled. I am besotted with him. I love him to bits. All my past pain pales into insignificance.

I am sure that Simon and I are going to be the best parents ever. I love feeding and bathing him although I have this fear deep inside me that something might go wrong or I might do something wrong. I am forever changing his clothes so that he looks pristine and beautiful at all times.

When Jay is four months old I am pregnant again. We don't know how we are going to manage financially, so I take an early morning cleaning job at Hackney Town Hall. I get up at four in the morning and leave Simon and Jay sleeping. By the time I arrive back home again at seven thirty AM, Simon is ready for work and Jay is ready for his next feed.

We don't have running water in our room, so I collect water in a bucket from the landing upstairs and boil hot water in a saucepan for cooking, washing and washing our clothes. We don't have a bathroom and we use the communal toilet on the ground floor. My dream is to be allocated a council flat and it seems that it will only happen if we move to a new town.

My relationship with Simon's parents improves after their first grandchild is born. I visit them two or three times during the week after I have cleaned my two rooms and finished any washing or ironing that needs doing. Simon's mother only works in the mornings, so I catch the bus to their flat in Finsbury Park. Simon's parents still don't think much of me, but they enjoy having their grandson around to visit. I usually arrive at their place by mid afternoon and wait for Simon to arrive there from work. Simon's mother makes us some tea and then we catch the bus home together.

Beth, my baby girl, is born in September 1969. Simon's parents look after Jay for a week while I am in hospital with Beth. Again Simon stays with me until he is asked to leave the delivery room and comes back in as soon as Beth is born. Although Beth is a smaller baby than Jay, I am in labour for over twenty-four hours. Beth feels more fragile than Jay and when I hold her in my arms, I feel a mixture of love and pleasure with my new baby daughter, who is so pretty and delicate just like a little doll. She has big blue eyes, a mop of dark hair and very fine features. I am also missing Jay and feeling afraid that I am not going to be able to manage two babies. I have a constant fear that something terrible is going to happen.
I still manage to visit Simon's parents' home during the week, but not as frequently as I did before Beth was born. Getting on and off buses with two babies is a struggle, money is also very tight and so I don't have money for bus fares. I visit my mother and Uncle Harry rarely. Uncle Harry

still whispers obscene sexual comments in my ear. On one occasion, my mother is in the kitchen and I am sitting in the living room with Beth in my arms. He says, "What happens when you're doing it with Simon, does he have an asthma attack? I bet he can't finish the job, can he?" I feel frozen inside and don't answer him.

When Beth is six months old we move from the slums of Hackney and far away from my mother and Uncle Harry. Wellingborough is a new town. We have a council house with three bedrooms, bathroom, running water and all the other amenities we need including a small garden for the children. So very different from the two rooms in Hackney.

My brother Dennis and his wife Janet move to Wellingborough with us. They live with us until they find a place of their own. Dennis and Simon don't have very much in common. My brother Dennis is well built and, like the men who he works with on the building sites, he likes a pint and loves to watch football. Simon, who is of a slight build, works as a shipping clerk in an office and hates all sports including football. Simon reads or occupies himself with crosswords if he has any spare time. The two men go out to work while Janet and I stay at home with Jay and Beth. Janet is of mixed race and Uncle Harry does not approve of her. He says to Dennis, "Have you thought about the consequences? If Janet has a baby it could be black." Dennis tells Uncle Harry to piss off and mind his own business. Dennis talking back to Uncle Harry in this way is very bold of him and an unusual way for Dennis to react. Dennis has always been very deferential towards Uncle Harry, especially in his teenage years.

I am a very anxious young mum and Janet, who is a bouncy tough nineteen year old, helps me with the children, who are both under two years old. She often gives me advice on how to look after Jay and Beth and helps me in the house. I can cook and clean all right but working out money, writing letters and paying bills are a nightmare! Dennis has similar problems around administration, so Simon and Janet deal with these issues. Dennis works as a carpenter and he can earn very good money. He also has some savings put away from an insurance payout from a motorcycle accident he had in his teens. This enables him to put a deposit on his own house.

Within six months Janet and my brother move out. Coping alone with the children leaves me feeling so scared. How am I going to manage? Simon can write the letters and pay the bills but he can't help me look after the children. Panic sweeps over me. I so want everything to be right. Jay and Beth need to look clean and to be seen as 'normal'. I am afraid that they may be seen as different from other children and I want them to be accepted by other children and adults in the area. I want them to be included and for other kids to want to play with them.

I feel such an odd and stupid woman and I fear that my children may be stigmatised because of me. I need help. I remember how it felt not to be accepted when I was a child. My experience of the children's homes and my unhappy childhood with the family come back and haunt me. I can hear my family, the psychiatrist and probation officers telling me over and over again that I must forget the past. I must just accept how things are. I tell myself, "Don't think about it. Then people won't think that you are crazy, strange or bad. You are just a little slow, not very bright, that's why you need help."
Simon cooks, helps around the house and is a good father to the children, but he is not a friend to me. We live together but we don't have much of a relationship.

Joe remains living in London with his wife and two children, Mathew and Tina. Joe is in a bad way, he is violent and he is often in trouble with the police. The children and I stay away from Joe and his family. He is seen as barking mad, no one ever crosses him. But this is how I have always known Joe. When we were growing up, Joe was such an angry boy who refused to be broken by Uncle Harry however hard he hit him or cruelly he baited him. Joe has total contempt for the authorities. His words often pop up in my mind, "Don't you ever tell those bastards anything, don't cry and don't tell them about our family or about what is going on."

I feel shy and I am not finding it easy to make friends in this new place. I feel scared when I am alone with Jay and Beth. I plead with Simon not to go to work, but to stay at home with the children and me. Simon goes to work. In fact, he also finds evening work, saying he needs to supplement our income.

I want to be a perfect mum for Jay and Beth, but when they fall ill or cry because they are overtired, I am at a loss to know what to do. I cuddle them a lot, I am fiercely protective of them if any of the neighbours criticise them, and I make sure the clothes that they are going to wear on the next day are clean and ironed and all sorted out the night before. Our G.P. tells me that I should control my children better, especially when Jay pulls things off his desk and runs madly around his office. I shrug my shoulders. I don't know what to do. I don't know how to stop Jay. I am at a loss to know where to turn.

The children and I are in the play park one day and one of the neighbours starts to talk to me. Her name is Linda. She is a single mum. Her little girl is called Kerry, she is a year or so older than Jay. Linda herself has just moved from London to Wellingborough and she seems as lonely as I am. A friendship starts to develop between us. As a way of subsidising her income, Linda starts childminding during the day. From the moment of meeting Linda I spend more time round at her house with Jay and Beth than I do in my own house. Simon works during the day and most evenings. He has found a job behind the bar in a Working Men's club. Linda advises me about almost anything to do with looking after Jay and Beth, even potty training Beth and what to do when either of the children becomes ill. I phone Linda and she says, "Bring them around here."

It is like a repeat of the children's home, only this time Linda takes Mummy Robins place. Even her height and build are similar. Linda is 5ft tall and her build is in proportion to her height. She has red short hair and a freckled face and pale blue eyes. I feel as if I can depend on her totally and I do so.

The children now both have blonde hair. Jay's hair falls into ringlets around his shoulders. He is a boisterous energetic little boy and keeps me busy. Beth is a very feminine little girl, she has the biggest bluest round eyes and she manages to get Jay and others to supply her needs. She is truly charming. Both my children are beautifully dressed and I am often stopped and asked if my children are models. I love them to bits and I am so proud. I love them in a way that I can never love Simon.

Simon and I see little of each other, this seems to suit him. He is a good father to our children. We don't really talk except about holidays or the children. He gives me security but not warmth or friendship.

I feel as if I am not in danger any longer, sometimes I even feel happy. In the summer months I play football on the green with Jay and the other kids who live on the estate and Linda and I go out shopping together. On Sunday lunch times we go with the children to the Working Men's

Club where Simon works. We never have much money so Linda and I will buy one round in order to get a glass each. Then we top up with pop and crisps that we have brought with us concealed in a bag.

Then there are moments when horrible memories come up quite unexpectedly. I am back there. I feel anxious and sad feelings sit in my tummy as if something dreadful is about to happen. Something is crying inside and memories of the children's home and of the sexual abuse by Uncle Harry are there. At these times I feel weird, almost mad, so confused. This voice inside my head says, "Don't say anything. Keep quiet." I feel as if I am walking about in a daze that no one ever seems to notice. This feeling can last for hours, sometimes days.

There are times when I go out for a short walk towards the school, a route that is well known to me. I am afraid to go alone to places that are not known to me. As I pass the trees, I remember the children's home and the words 'If you go down to the woods today' come to mind. I begin to hurry along and I think of something else.

Jay and Beth start school. I avoid having contact with their teachers because my vocabulary is poor and I feel stupid and ashamed. I pray that Jay and Beth will not feel ashamed of me, so I leave it to Simon or Linda to talk to the teachers on parents evening. I wait for them by the school gate.

There are times when we are short of money. Linda agrees to look after the children and I go out to work, just for a few weeks. I find work in a clothes factory that makes school uniforms. The factory makes skirts, trousers and school blazers. I lie about my ability to use a sewing machine, and I am asked to sew on the arms of the blazers. The supervisor shows me once or twice what to do and to my surprise I pick it up.

Simon begins to have doubts about where he is working. He says the money is poor as are prospects of promotion. He looks for other work in the area but is not successful. Also Linda has met a man and spends most of her time with him these days. I still go to see her for a chat from time to time but our friendship has changed. Simon suggests that we apply for a council house exchange and move back to London. This seems like a good option. We plan to move back to the area in which we have both grown up.

We exchange properties with a family who live in a flat on the fifth floor just off Brecknock Road in Islington. We are a bus journey away from both Simon's parents and my mother and Uncle Harry and the children's new school is just a few yards away from our new flat.

We move in the September of 1974. I can't remember any of the details about moving from Wellingborough to Islington I don't know why but it's a complete blank.

CHAPTER SIX
HOPE FOR THE FUTURE

My world is falling apart. I have made a dreadful mistake returning to London. What have I done? Everything is collapsing around me and I feel so frightened. I don't know anyone. I am so scared.

On my return to London from Wellingborough I have several severe breakdowns, which force me to have inpatient psychiatric treatment. I continue to tell my story over and over again in a most incoherent way, with constant repetition of the details of the sexual abuse, to Maria, Pat and other day centre staff. I am frequently in and out of Friern Barnet Hospital. Maria and the day centre staff are concerned that my mental health is deteriorating rather than improving. The psychiatrist tells Maria that I will be in and out of psychiatric hospitals for most of my life so damaging was my childhood.

I am feeling guilty and very distressed. Jay and Beth stay at the children's home every time that I am hospitalised. I have refused to take my prescribed medication. I flush it down the toilet, saying, "This isn't what I need. I don't want to be so drugged up that I can't function. I feel and appear like a zombie."

Yet at the same time, I want the flood of memories to stop swamping me. My memories come into my head and then they are discharged. It is like verbal diarrhoea. I can't stop talking about it.

Maria talks to me about referring me to a therapeutic hospital called the Henderson Hospital. She tells me that I will have to stay as an inpatient for ten months to a year, and that the hospital doesn't use prescribed drugs. The treatment involves talking through my problems in a group.

As an attempt to let me know that I am believed, the social workers go to see my mother. On the understanding that there will be no prosecutions, my mother and brother Joe admit that what I have told them was true. My brother Dennis denies his part in the abuse, which causes me no great surprise. He never accepted any responsibility for his part in things when we were young. Others always took the blame. He and his wife have written to tell me how despicable I am for allowing my children to go into care. From that day to this I have no further contact with Dennis or his family.

I discover that the Henderson Hospital is for people who don't improve or fit into conventional psychiatric hospital or people who have committed criminal offences. They are perceived as having a personality disorder which causes disturbed behaviour.

Maria, my social worker, takes me there. I don't know what to expect. I arrive and am taken into a huge hall where there are people sitting around in a circle. I am told that this is a group interview and that some of the people are patients and there are also three members of staff, a psychiatrist, a nurse who doesn't wear a uniform, and a therapist. I can't tell who the patients are and who the members of staff are. I feel very scared. So scared that I don't think too much about what the questions are. It is as if someone else from inside of me takes me over and answers their questions. When I arrive back home I can't recall what questions I was asked.

I wait for a letter to arrive to say whether I will or won't be accepted. I am afraid that if I'm not accepted, I will be unable to pull myself out of this terrible mess that I am in, I will lose Jay and Beth, and that thought is unbearable.

I don't have to wait long before I receive a letter saying that I have been accepted for treatment at the Henderson.

My children are placed in another children's home, different to the one they were in before. It is explained to both Simon and me that the change is due to the children's stay being seen as long term, longer than they have stayed in care previously. Simon is going to have Jay and Beth at home at weekends and when I have settled down at the Henderson I can also join them for weekend visits.

The Henderson Hospital is a run down old building. The part of the hospital that is occupied by the Henderson is still standing but the rest is derelict. There is a run down old kitchen. A community room, with old damaged chairs to sit on, is the biggest room there. This is where all the big meetings take place. The women's ward is at one end of the building and two men's wards are at the other end, near the front entrance. The wards consist of rows of cubicles made out of plywood.
For the first few weeks I sit and watch what is going on. I am too terrified to talk or make any contribution to any of the groups. I only speak when I am directly asked something. Some of the patients who are here seem rough and much tougher than me.
My day starts with the big meeting in the main hall, which is called the nine thirty meeting. Everyone is expected to be here: all the patients, the four psychiatrists who work here and the nurses and therapists that are on duty. The meeting breaks up and the patients form small groups.

At first I attend a small group that all new patients attend for the first four weeks. After that time I join a small group that is lead by a Spanish psychiatrist, two nurses, one therapist and a training therapist. The first thing that I notice is that all the patients are male except me. I put my head down and hope that I am not noticed. Towards the end of the small group session I am asked to choose an activity group for the afternoon. I am told that there is a drama group, an art therapy group, a woodwork group and a group who prepare and cook the evening meal for patients and staff. I choose to work in the kitchen.

During the evenings there is a ward meeting or a psychodrama group. If there are no groups, then my time is my own, unless a fight breaks out or some one has freaked out, then a ward meeting is called. The big-three, who are three patients that have been elected by the community to represent the patients, chair the nine thirty morning meeting and meet with the staff that are on duty at nine thirty in the evening. Together they draw up an agenda based on the events of the day, which is taken to the meeting the following morning.

The morning meetings are huge, it is difficult for me to get inside the door and sit down, let alone say anything. Anyone who has broken any of the rules has to explain themselves to the rest of the community. A vote is then taken to decide if they can stay or whether they should leave the hospital. A young guy has set light to a big dustbin just outside the kitchen door. He hasn't been at the Henderson for long and has done this sort of thing before, both since his arrival and before he came to the Henderson. The head psychiatrist says to everyone in the meeting, "Do we want to push this man to start more fires?" I guess he means that the pressure of being at the Henderson makes this guy act out in this way. He is asked to leave. Any crimes that are committed by patients are reported to the police. During my stay here at the Henderson two men are arrested, one for sexually assaulting a fourteen-year-old girl and the other for burglary.

I am cooking the evening meal with three other patients during the afternoon cookery group. Everything seems to be going fine, when there is a sudden eruption from

Maureen, one of the women in the group. She screams and shouts at all the people around her, pots and pans are thrown and just about everything she can lay her hands on is smashed. Then she pulls out a razor and starts cutting herself across her arms. She is shouting obscenities about her mother. "Fucking bitch. Don't you keep watching me and telling me what to do. There isn't anything that I can do right according to you. Shut up, just shut up. I fucking hate you."

Maureen is taken to the local general hospital for stitches to her arms. When she returns to the Henderson hospital a ward meeting is called. She talks through what caused her outburst and what effect it has on the people who were around her. Maureen talks about her relationship with her mother and how controlling her mother was. Cooking in the kitchen reminded Maureen of how her mother used to go on and on at her until she couldn't take it any more. Maureen does manage to gain some insight into herself and the build-up to her outburst.

A few days later in the same cooking group, I am standing gazing into space when one of the nurses runs over to me and lifts my hand off the hot electric cooker plate. I am completely unaware that my hand is burning. As the nurse dresses my hand I say in a whisper, "I'm sorry." When I join my morning small group, the psychiatrist starts to question my choice of activity group in the afternoon. I say, "I chose the cookery group because I think that is what I am good at."

The psychiatrist persuades me to join in the art therapy group, and he says, "Isn't it time for you to play and have fun?" I continue with that group until I leave the Henderson.

The psychiatrist and others in the small group begin to encourage me to talk about the clothes that I am wearing:

a straight skirt, flat shoes and a plain baggy jumper. It is pointed out to me that I dress like a woman in her forties rather than a twenty six year old. It is interpreted by the psychiatrist that I have become my mother, and was that the person that I am cutting when I cut my arms?

This interpretation stuns me. I physically feel my body move as if someone has jolted me. It has a profound effect on me. I never again deliberately cut or burn myself.

Over time my style of dress changes. I start to dress in jeans, with a jumper or a T-shirt, more like teenagers would have dressed when I was a teenager.

I began to see that there are lots of different people at the Henderson and from very different backgrounds. The patients that I know most about are the ones in my small group. Shaun, an older man, is a compulsive gambler. He gambles all his money away and then gets involved in fraud. He has been to prison on several occasions, but this is not a deterrent for him. In fact, he feels safe in prison, being held securely in his prison cell by four walls. Shaun comes to the conclusion that his gambling is about gaining power through wealth, but he never keeps any of the money that he wins. Tony is another guy that I become friendly with. Tony's mother had dressed him like a girl for the first five years of his life and she kept him in the house and didn't allow him to play with other children. It was only when he started school that his mother acknowledged that he was a boy and dressed him like a boy. Tony has been in and out of psychiatric hospitals for years, and I think he is quite crazy. If he thinks that anyone is looking at him or suggests that he looks effeminate in any way, he flies into uncontrollable rages and threatens to hit people.

An interpretation is made about my friendship with Shaun and Tony. One of the therapists says, "I think that while you have been here, they have become a replacement for your brothers." This prompts me to talk about my brothers and my place in the family. At the bottom, they were always the cowboys and I was always the Indian, in other words the underdog.

Two women join the small group that I am in, and I find it difficult to relate to either of them easily. Anne seems to come from a perfect family. She was an only child. Her parents have adopted and fostered many children. Anne cuts herself savagely. She is sullen and rarely talks to anyone. Anne's mother is invited in for family meetings but this doesn't seem to make any difference to Anne's self-hatred.

Anita, the other girl in my small group, admits to hitting her little girl quite badly. Her child has been taken away from her. Anita readily talks about herself, her childhood and her little girl. She comes to understand that her violence towards her own daughter is a repetition of what she herself has suffered as a child. Anita was in callipers as a small child. Her parents punished her and other children, excluded her and laughed at her.

I am asked if I can understand Anita's behaviour. I stubbornly say, "No, no, I can't. I can't understand how anyone can beat up a child." I can feel a rage building up inside of me, just thinking about it. I storm out of the group.

When I feel this way I take myself into the derelict part of the old hospital where I can smash all the windows that I can find, or I hit a ball with a bat, hard against the wall until I am exhausted.

I am at the Henderson for a couple of months before I start to go home for weekends. I collect the children from the children's home on Friday evening. Beth seems able to reach out to her carers. She is very close to John, her key worker. When I arrived to collect the children this Friday, I found Beth sitting on John's lap, giggling as she combed

John's bushy ginger beard. Jay is standing close by them watching. He laughs with them but doesn't show a need to be close to anyone other than his mum and dad. A senior member of staff talks to me before I leave about what I have planned and what we might do as a family. Jay and Beth are excited and pleased to see both Simon and me. We go to the park or stay at home for most of the weekend. Money is short and we can't visit Simon's family. They are not very pleased with what is happening. As for my mother and Uncle Harry, I stay away.

I leave my house on Sunday afternoon at about four o'clock to return to the Henderson. Simon takes the children to school on Monday morning, and a member of staff from the children's home collects Jay and Beth from school on Monday evening.

I hate leaving Jay and Beth. A pang of guilt tugs at me. I look at their little faces and see their confusion. Jay tells me how he looks after Beth, "I will look after her, mummy. I stay with her and make sure that she is alright." Such a big boy at only eight years old. Beth's teacher from school visits Beth at the children's home and both Beth and Jay tell me how they look forward to daddy getting them ready for bed and reading to them before they go to sleep. Simon visits the children most weekday evenings. He goes there from work.

In my small group, I tell them, "I miss Jay and Beth so much. I can't bear leaving them behind all the time. It feels so wrong and I know how much it hurts them. I am their mother, I should be with them.
Dr Diego says, "But you really can't do that at the moment, Pam. You are not ready. If you take them out of care and you need to return to hospital because you are not coping, that will cause more harm and confusion. You are doing

the best thing for your children by being here and working on your problems."

I miss Jay and Beth terribly. I feel that they need to be cared for in a loving family. But I know that Dr Diego is right, I can't do that until I have sorted myself out. However, illogically I cling to the belief that I should be looking after them and feel bad about not doing so.

I'm home for a weekend. On Saturday I catch the 253 bus to Stamford Hill. I pass Manor House tube station and the flat that I grew up in. I feel very weird, it is as if I am transported back in time, while I also remain where I am, but looking in at my past life. My past life is like a play being performed on stage, with me as a member of the audience. I don't tell anyone at the hospital about this incident. They may think that I am crazy.

After a while I become conscious of the scars on my arms and I start to cover my arms up so that people won't see them. The psychiatrist asks me if I have ever thought about having a skin craft. He refers me to St. George's hospital.

I go to see the consultant, he sees me in front of about ten students. He looks at one of the students and says, "What do you think? Should I put her on the waiting list?"

He looks back at me and says, "I don't think so, why should public money be wasted on you? How soon will it be before you do this again?"

I feel so ashamed and small. When I return to the Henderson the psychiatrist is very annoyed when he discovers what the consultant has said to me. He came back to me a week later and tells me that I am on the waiting list for a skin craft.

The art therapy group starts to bring me out of myself. I am and was never good at drawing or painting but I am encouraged to play with the paints and, after people in the group have finished their work, we talk about our paintings. Mine vary from missing my children to the crying child that I feel inside myself. Once I painted the faces of three children with tears running down their faces. We don't just paint. We also have a go at pottery, just for fun.

It is almost Christmas time. We are making our own Christmas cards. My pictures are of perfect loving families huddled together by a Christmas tree. The art therapist points out that, although that's what Christmas cards portray, not every one experiences a loving family. This is my fantasy.

The doctors at the Henderson have invited my mother and my brothers to attend a family meeting. My mother and oldest brother Joe agree to come along. The meeting is set for 11am on Tuesday. I leave my small group at 10.45am and wait for my mother and brother to arrive. I wait in the front hall until 12.30pm and still hope that they will turn up, saying to myself, "Maybe they have been held up in traffic, or the train has broken down."

By 1pm the staff say that they are sorry but they feel sure my mother will not come now. I return to my room feeling ashamed and stupid. How can I have a mother who doesn't care about what happens to me? I sit on my bed and stare out of the window.

One of the therapists comes into my room to check that I am O.K. I say that I am. It is a shock to me that she came to enquire about me. Members of staff never have one-to-one contact with patients.

I stay in my room until the next day and when I join my small group the therapist who came to see me in my room says that my room surprises her. She says, "It is so bare." I ask her what she means. She says, "There are no pictures on your wall and your room is bare and empty, you have no personal possessions".

I say, "The room represents me, empty and worthless."

Simon and I are invited to join in a couples group that meets at the Henderson once a fortnight on Monday evenings. When we first join the group there is another couple besides Simon and myself, there is also a psychiatrist and the art therapist from my art therapy group. In the first few sessions the psychiatrist concentrates on the other couple. He occasionally asks Simon and me to comment on the other couple's problems or what is being discussed in the session. It is almost like an introduction to what is expected of Simon and me when it comes to our turn to look at our relationship. The other couple leaves the couples group. The male partner has finished his treatment at the Henderson

Simon and I talk about how we first met and how we both agreed for me to get pregnant so that we could marry. Simon says, "I was under twenty one and I knew that my parents would never agree unless Pam was pregnant with my child. I never felt trapped. I also wanted to leave home at that time."
Simon talks about his envy towards his younger brother and how after five years of being an only child, he felt left out and rejected by his parents when James was born. He felt that his mother favoured his younger brother.
From what I have seen of the family together, I think that Simon has a point. Simon feels very bitter about this and it comes to light that there are times when Simon lets this experience affect how he relates to our son Jay, as if Jay is the favoured son over himself.
In the couples group we talk and explore how we communicate with each other. It is pointed out that we spent very little time together throughout the years that we lived in Wellingborough. Simon worked all day and then would work as a barman in the evenings. I also took up work at one point, working weekends as a cook in an old people's home. We rarely had time together as a family.

Simon's resentment towards me becomes very evident. He says, "I preferred it that way. I was happy to continue to do my own thing."

He looks directly at me and says, "I don't love you, and I never have".

His statement shocks me. I sit there and say nothing.

Simon continues to talk about his anger towards me, how I have hurt him and let him down. He is unhappy with our sexual relationship. He says, "You are frigid and cold and I have only stayed in this relationship with you because of the children."

I can't recall the session ending. I feel as if I have been kicked in the stomach.

As we leave the room Simon cuddles me and says that he is sorry.

We continue the couples group and we talk further about our sexual relationship. I admit my dislike for sexual contact. I want Simon to cuddle me rather than us having sex together. We are both encouraged to spend more time together, to talk about what we are feeling rather than keeping our feelings to ourselves. We also look at how we care for Jay and Beth and our relationship with them. I come to understand how we need to function as a family unit, and how both the children are going to need our support in readjusting when we are back home together as a family.

I am becoming stronger, more able to talk both in the small groups and in the large community meeting. I am elected by the community to become one of the big three. To my amazement I can not only talk in this group but also lead the morning meetings.

I am beginning to plan the end of my stay at the Henderson hospital with the Henderson staff and my social worker. One of the nurses tells me, "You have done so well, Pam. Although you were offered a place at the Henderson, you were not expected to last longer than two weeks because at that time you were too fragile."

Maria, my social worker, has left and Penny, my new social worker, visits me at the Henderson on a regular basis three or four months before leaving the Henderson. It feels strange meeting with Penny as it is the policy at the Henderson for patients to talk to members of staff in a group setting, never on a one to one basis. When Penny visits she feels like an extension of the Henderson staff, she wants to know how I am feeling and what thoughts I am having and also thoughts about my past. She says that when I leave the Henderson she will be there as a social worker for the family and she can also offer me weekly counselling sessions. I begin to feel very close to her as well as feeling dependent upon seeing her.

Before the children can come home, Simon and I are invited to a meeting at the children's home. When we arrive there a member of staff is waiting for us. The staff member introduces us to a psychiatrist, who tells us that he is representing Islington Social Services. Simon and I sit down and both Jay and Beth stand beside us. The psychiatrist says, without any introduction to what the meeting is about, "I don't know whether it is in the best interests of Jay and Beth to return to their family home, it might be better for us to think about adoption."

Jay clings to me and says whilst crying and stamping his feet, "No mummy, no mummy, I want to come home with you." Beth starts to cry and holds on to her dad's leg.

I am stunned as is Simon. I ask, "What is going on?" The psychiatrist says, "Do you think that the children will ever go back into care if they go home with you now?"

I explain about all the work we did at the Henderson. "I have worked hard and we attended a couples' group, during my stay at the Henderson."

Simon says we have learnt a lot about ourselves and we have learnt about what Jay and Beth will need from us when we get back home together as a family.

It is decided that the children can come home with us. They are coming home this weekend and arrangements are made for them to return home for good on the following Friday.

As we leave the room another member of staff takes Simon, Beth, Jay and myself into the kitchen and says, "I am so sorry about what has happened. No one, including the staff, expected that to happen."

She says, "I think that the psychiatrist was testing both of you out to see what your reaction was going to be."

I am so pleased that Simon and I have passed the test.

The children are home and we seem to settle back to normal life again quite quickly. I get myself an early morning cleaning job, the children continue to go to school and Simon goes to work. I clean the house and cook the evening meal. I am very keen for the children to get a lot of new clothes. The clothes they have returned home with are tatty and they don't have much to wear. We re-establish contact with Simon's parents and plan a family holiday with them for the following year. It is important to me that Jay and Beth have what other kids have and family holidays come somewhere near to the top of my list.

Penny, our social worker, visits us all at home and she starts to see me at her office for weekly counselling sessions. The counselling sessions are going well. Penny starts to reflect back some of my behaviour towards her. In the session she says, "You are like a young child. I almost feel that what you need is to be like a small child with me."

I am aware of feelings of love and dependency towards Penny. I turn up at her office unannounced, sometimes wet because I have walked in the rain from Seven Sisters Road to the Archway, where her office is, without a coat or anything to keep me dry. I kick up a fuss when she says that she can't see me.

In our next session she tells me that she can't see me on my own again. She says, "This isn't your fault. I am not blaming you. The Henderson has warned me not to stir up your feelings around your mother and I think that is what I have done."

Penny pauses and takes an intake of breath before she continues, "I am in training as a counsellor and I have taken on something that I can't handle."

This was like a bolt from the blue. Penny had dropped a bombshell on me from a great height. I sit there in numb silence.

Before leaving her office she says that she has arranged for Simon and me to meet with her and another counsellor for family sessions.

Two weeks later we are at the family meeting that Penny has arranged. Both Simon and I are offered a cup of coffee. I feel an un-containable rage swelling up inside my tummy. I throw my cup at the wall, shouting obscenities at Penny, "You fucking bitch, you set this up to make me look like a fucking idiot. I am not staying here with you because you are just like the rest of them." I storm out of the room.

That was the end of the family sessions. Shortly afterwards I turn up at Penny's office again. I am still feeling angry and that I have been misunderstood and unfairly treated. I demand to see her. She sends a message out via the receptionist. She won't see me. I plead with the receptionist that I need her to explain to Penny that I don't know what I have done wrong. Penny comes out of her office. She says, "I am trying to refer you to another counsellor but that is going to take time."

Penny returns to her office and closes her office door behind her.

"She hasn't told me what I have done wrong," I scream at the receptionist, "and I'm not leaving until she does."

The receptionist threatens to call the police if I don't leave. This makes me even angrier and more distressed. I kick a small coffee table over and throw a chair across the room. The police are called. As I see the police arriving, I run out of the office and along an open balcony that is about one and a half stories high. The police corner me and I climb onto the wall of the balcony in an attempt to jump off and get away. I am wrestled to the ground and taken to the police station where I am seen by a doctor. I am still shouting, "It isn't my fault and I don't know what I have done wrong."

I am sectioned and taken to the local psychiatric hospital. It is late evening by the time I arrive there. They give me medication to calm me down but waves of panic sweep over me. I have to go home to Jay and Beth. I keep leaving my room pleading and trying to explain it to the male nurse who is on duty. He says, "Yes, yes," as he guides me back to my room.

On the fourth time of bothering him he twists my arm up my back and slams me against a wall. He then pushes me into my room and says, "Stay there."

I stay in my room until the early morning. As I creep out of my room, I find that the main door on the ward has been left unlocked. It has probably been left unlocked for the day staff that are coming on duty.

I am sedated and I wobble as I walk down the stairs and out of the hospital. I can't make it all the way back to my house. I make my way to Pat's house, the social worker from the day centre. Pat lives closer to the hospital. I tell

Pat everything that has happened, including the incident with the male nurse. She explains to me, "You must to go back to the hospital, Pam. You are under a section and if you go home the police will arrest you and that might be in front of Jay and Beth. You don't want that to happen, do you? Come on, I will go back to the hospital with you."

Pat comes back to the hospital with me. She talks to the doctor on her own. Pat leaves the room and the doctor calls me into his office. He keeps asking how high the wall that I was going to jump off was. I say, "I am not very good at describing heights in feet and inches but it wasn't that high and I was not intending to hurt myself. I just wanted to get away from the police."

He asks me about the allegation that I have made about the male nurse. I tell him what happened. He says, "Do you want to go home?"

I understand what he means and say, "Alright, nothing happened."

The section is lifted and I go home.

Much to my dismay and horror the story is written up in the local newspaper implying that I was suicidal, attempting to jump off a tower block and that the policewoman was a heroine. This is all untrue. I protest, but to no avail. My fear is that I already have a bad reputation with my neighbours. They see me as mad. This will simply confirm it for them.

Pat suggests that after finishing my cleaning job, it will help me if I return to the daycentre which I had attended before going to the Henderson until a counsellor is found for me.

THERAPY WITH HELLE
CHAPTER SEVEN

It's not fair, why won't anyone work with me? They work with all those other people who have parents. Why do they get everything and I get nothing? I wish this awful pain would go away.

I am referred to various counselling agencies but they all say that I am too damaged or they feel that they don't have enough experience to work with someone like me. Other agencies tell me that they have very long waiting lists. I go to the Women's Therapy Centre, for an assessment. They are based near to Beth and Jay's School, but they also tell me that they have a long waiting list. I can not and will not take no for an answer. I am really feeling angry and frustrated; it seems to me that this is a repeat of my childhood; nobody wants to work with the likes of me.

Penny has referred me to the London Centre for Psychotherapy. I am soon to meet Helle.

Helle, a softly spoken woman, wears her grey hair in a bun. She is very slender and looks like a kind woman. She asks me to explain what is wrong and how she can help. Feelings start to bubble up inside me. I tell her how unfair this world is. Helle slows me down, she talks to me in a quiet soothing voice. This lessens the intensity of my feelings.

Helle tells me very firmly that if we are going to work together there are rules and boundaries that I am expected to keep within. She says, "You must not smash my windows or smash-up anything in my consulting room or anything in this building. I don't own this room, I rent it and you won't be allowed to come here if you do anything like that." She went on to say, "If you get angry you must not hit me or throw anything at me and if you get into trouble outside of my consulting room, I will not be able to help you, Pam. You are going to have to work out your difficulties here in this room, verbally, not out there."

I can't afford much money in terms of paying for therapy. Simon doesn't earn that much and I am paid even less at my two and a half hour early morning cleaning job. Helle charges me what she has to pay for her room rent at L.C.P. with the understanding that Helle's charges will increase in line with my earnings.

Having found someone who will work with me, I feel a tremendous need to communicate and be understood. However, I find it very difficult to make this woman understand what I am trying to find words for. I feel speedy, excited and frustrated because the response that I want from Helle is not there. I begin to test out most of the rules. I refuse to leave at the end of my session. I get so angry with her when she tells me that my session has finished that I take her clock out of the consulting room with me and refuse to give it back to her. I say, "I want to smash it into small pieces."

Helle gives up asking me to give it back to her and returns to her consulting room with her next patient. I leave it, intact, outside her room.

In the next session I become very frustrated and angry with her when she doesn't understand me and in a flash of rage I kick over her coffee table and run out of the session.

I return home and try to behave as if everything is normal. I collect Jay and Beth from school and cook the evening meal. I feel like a robot. If I keep myself busy cleaning and concentrating on tasks around the home, I can cut off from what I am feeling.

It's when I go to bed that my anger starts to rage out of my control. I get up in the middle of the night and pace up and down. I make my way onto the street where there is a pay phone and I phone Helle. I tell her that she does not understand and doesn't care about me and I feel that it is all very unfair.

Over the next few sessions I gradually learn that, despite Helle's patience, she remains firm around the boundaries that she has laid down. This helps me to feel secure. She stays, she doesn't disintegrate and she doesn't reject me. My rage and confusion lift a bit and we begin to understand the symbolic meaning of my acting out as a way of communicating about my teenage rebellion against my mother.

I become aware of deeper feelings, a longing for the sort of mothering that I have never received but tried to give my children when they were small. I ask Helle if we could pretend that she is my mother.

She is very hesitant. She asks me if I have a sexuality problem. I repeat over and over again that these feelings are different from sexual feelings. Helle says, "Pam, play therapy is commonly used with small children and I think that it might work for you."

We agree to try this way of working but Helle tells me, "This will only work under very strict rules. You have to behave as an adult between sessions. When you are in the consulting room you can regress but only here, then you can go back to being a child and we will try to understand what is going on."

I understand that I have to keep to this agreement but it is very difficult for me.

I am still kicking Helle's table over on occasions. I decide to lie down on her couch in an attempt to stop this impulse. This makes me feel small and helpless. I feel as if I don't have enough power in my legs to damage anything. I also

find that without actually doing anything I can tell mummy Helle what I want to do. "I want to kick my legs."
Helle asks why I want to kick.
I say, "It's not fair everyone else has a family and I don't".
A rage swells up inside my tummy and I tell Mummy Helle that "IT is coming up through my tummy. IT always comes when I feel it's not fair and others have all that I want. IT is a very strong and angry monster."
Mummy Helle asks me what colour my monster is. "It's green and very strong."
Helle says that my green monster won't hurt me because she is there. She holds my hand and I feel safe as if I am sitting on her lap. After lying very still, feeling held, I try to peep at mummy Helle, just for a moment, not any longer as I think that she might shatter.
This sort of play continues for some weeks until my green monster becomes less frequent and violent. Towards the end of the session I sit up and Helle and I talk adult to adult.
I am never able to look at Helle during my therapy session, except momentarily.

Helle is going away for a week. I fear that Helle will disintegrate and disappear. This fear increases. I have images of little Pam waving to an aeroplane. There is a sad feeling in my tummy and Helle is going to fall down from the sky. At nights my dreams become very vivid, with walls crashing down and the sky caving in. When Helle comes back from her holiday I talk about how close I had felt to Mummy Robins in the children's home where I stayed from two until almost seven years old.

Between my sessions I phone Helle, by arrangement. I phone her once a day except on Saturdays. I don't have a phone at home. I use the public phone on my way to work at seven in the morning and on Sundays I get up before

Simon or the children wake up and use the public phone in the street where we live. On this occasion there is someone else waiting to use the phone. I can see her and I turn my face and pretend that I don't. The woman starts to bang on the door telling me to hurry up. I feel like a baby who has been distracted from feeding. I turn and open the door of the phone booth and scream and shout at her like a mad woman.

I phone Helle just before Christmas. She asks, "What would little Pam like for Christmas?"
I said, "Mummy, my monster wants a bottle!"
Mummy Helle replies; "Little Pam wants a nice drink of water? Very well, very soon now."
When Mummy Helle gives me a bottle, I feel warm inside. My monster is calm and mummy turns into beautiful patterns of different shades of light and colours.
I ask Mummy Helle why she keeps turning into a pattern. I draw pictures for her and tell her that I love her; I love my mummy lots and lots and lots. She tells me stories of the joys and fears of little Pam living with her mummy.

A lot of images come up. Long rows of cots. Children playing outside the window. Trees and their leaves, and sometimes I see a very little Pam sitting in her pushchair outside, around the corner from where the children are playing. I feel that I have no legs and that I can't play with the others. I sit and watch the leaves on the tree making patterns. I feel miserable and dead inside.
After a while the peeping at Mummy Helle develops into games of hide-and-seek. This reminds me of playing hide-and-seek with Mummy Robins in the children's home. I feel a great deal of pleasure at being found.

Helle buys me a doll to play with. I pull off its legs and drop it on the floor. Then I put myself onto the floor and cover myself with a blanket instead of playing with the doll. I feel a tingling in my bottom. I think that I have been naughty. The pleasure feeling from having drunk my bottle has disappeared. I am alone with no legs. There is nothing except a baby inside my tummy, which I am rocking. Mummy Helle keeps calling my name softly, "Pam, Pam where are you?"

I wait for mummy Helle to pick me up. She doesn't. I throw myself against her legs and hold her hand.

As I rest my head on her knees, she strokes my hair. I am now able to tell her of the flashbacks. I am sitting in a cot, I have no legs and a woman is cross with me and lays me down. I can hear children playing outside. Then I see a long corridor and people in white coats coming towards me. I stretch my arms out to be picked up, but they always walk past.

Mummy Helle pulls me up to sit on the couch and puts an arm around me. During the nights that follow this session I wake up sweating, having dreamt that I was back in the corridor with people walking past me, and the walls closing in on me.

It takes a long time to reconstruct the events behind this re-enactment. We think that some time around the age of eighteen months old I was in a very distressed state, unable to walk or talk and reluctant to eat. Maybe some change occurred and the world I had known disappeared. Perhaps I was moved from the infants to the toddlers' part of the residential nursery where I was placed as a small baby.

Helle starts to introduce biscuits into my session. The bottle continues on and off for some time with Helle playing with me as the big girl. This brings up memories of playing with Mummy Robins at the children's home where I was transferred from the nursery. I learnt to walk and talk again.

I say to Helle how painful it was to lose Ruthy who was "choosed" by new parents. "No one ever choosed me," I say in a small voice.

I tell Helle how I remember being introduced to my mother by Uncle Harry. I don't understand how but I knew him before knowing her. With great pain I recall how the boys already knew her. She must have visited them regularly but did not know me (three years old?).

Memories of when my mother visited the children's home start to come up. I tell Helle about wanting to hide away. I say, "I did not want to be with her or Uncle Harry."

Angry and frightening feelings arise inside my tummy.

"I am afraid that they will see how I am feeling."

I can see me in the woods. Eerie scary feelings swamp me. A song plays in my mind. "If you go down to the woods today, be sure of a big surprise."

I push the song away out of my mind.

My legs want to kick but instead they collapse. There is nowhere to go, Mummy Robins will have nothing to do with me and Joe is angry with me, he wants to be with his mum. Reliving this with Helle, I feel confused and disoriented. I ask Helle, "Why would my mother want me home? She hates me."

I recall the times when I am forced to go home to Uncle Harry's house. I see myself hiding under a table where I sit and rock.

I relive this period of my life with Helle, and I feel full of trapped, lingering, crying pains in my diaphragm.

I tell Helle how it feels when my mother takes us home from the children's home, how I don't feel that I belong. "My bedroom is the sofa in the front room. Why can't I have a bedroom like my brothers?" "I hate it here. Mum is always ill, she vomits and has diarrhoea. Uncle Harry says that it is our fault and he hits us with 'Uncle Jack', the stick that stands in the corner."

Reflecting with Helle on this period during therapy, I can see how provocative Joe and I were on one or two occasions. There were times when we smashed the stick into pieces and waited for the consequences. On other occasions we showed our resentment towards Uncle Harry. Once, when a bonfire was lit at the camp, Joe was asked to pass some water to put the fire out; he handed over paraffin in an attempt to destroy Uncle Harry. All three of us ran and ran to avoid the repercussions.

I tell Helle how Uncle Harry was determined to knock us into shape. But Joe and I are equally determined not to let him see any hurt or pain in us.
I explain, "There was an unwritten code in our family that you did not tell your school friends or anyone else what happened at home and we didn't show that bastard that he had hurt us."

I talk to Helle about Uncle Harry and the sexual abuse. I go back there. "I feel this awful physical pain when he pushed his penis into my anus."
As my mind wanders I tell her, "It is disgusting, I feel that my body is out of shape. I look at myself in the mirror that is in my mother's bedroom. To me my breasts look an odd shape, huge and horrible where he has pulled at them, and it looks as if he has pushed my vagina forward, as if his penis had pushed everything down there forward.
"Did he make my body look like that?" I ask. I am now back in the room with Helle.
Helle reassures me, "You have given birth to two children, Pam, and if there was anything wrong with your body, the doctors would have noticed."

Helle's words make sense but my dislike of my body continues.

I recall a time when I refused Uncle Harry's sexual advances. I begin to tell Helle about it. I go back there in my mind, "He is caning me and the beating is getting more and more violent. I can't feel anything. I am not in pain when the stick strikes my bare bottom. I feel a rage in my tummy and I mumble at him, "Dirty old bastard." I say it in a whisper to Helle.
"He loses his usual self-control, he is hitting me harder and quicker, my mother pulls him away from me. I adjust my clothes as I say in a hurt angry voice,"I hate you, I hate you both."
My mother starts to punch into me, telling me to shut up.
I manage to get out of the front door. I am trembling with rage. I run down the balcony, jump down one flight of stairs, then another, then the third, the fourth. I think that I am going to burst with rage and energy. I jump over a fence, cross the road, then run and run until I have reached the swing park. I climb over the fence. I am now on some green land. I feel safe. I spend the night there watching the trees and their leaves. My anger dies down. I feel a sad crying pain in my tummy. The trees continue to offer me sanctuary. I spend hours alone at our local green area. Here my gentler feelings are given some space, though there are never any tears."
I tell Helle how I hate that world and all the adults that lived in it.

I talk to Helle about the sadness that I feel when I look back on my relationship with my two brothers, "I loved and respected Joe and when our friendship started to turn sour I felt so betrayed by both of them. The sexual play with them turned violent and they taunted me when Uncle Harry was making me sit in the corner."

I couldn't understand how or why they could kick me as they passed saying, "Slag, no good slag."

I tell Helle, "I am back there."

"Don't let them say that. I'm not a slag, don't let them tell me that, I plead to my mother, but she refuses to protect me. She starts to slap and punch me around my head. But my brother's betrayal hurts me much more than my mother's beatings. I feel so confused. Joe hates me. After the punishment period inflicted by Uncle Harry is over, Joe comes home late. It's night time and he comes to my bed and wakes me up. He tells me all about what he has been doing with his friends, he tells me that he loves me and asks me to play sexual games with him.

He says, "You pretend that you are a striptease model."

I do and it excites him, and then he gets me to masturbate him.

When I tell Joe about what Uncle Harry is doing he says, "It doesn't matter. I'm doing it too and it isn't harming you."

Joe doesn't come to my bed tonight and I wake up with Dennis lying on top of me. He says, "Lie still, it won't take long."

He pushes his penis up and down my tummy until he has climaxed. He roles off of me and returns to his own bedroom. Sometimes I lie awake waiting for one of them to come into the sitting room. It is better than being on my own. I hate it when no one will talk to me and during the periods of punishment I am sent to Coventry. That's what Uncle Harry calls it. He says, "When people have been bad they get punished. I am sending you to Coventry. Do you understand no one is to talk to her?" By now I am twelve or thirteen.

I tell Helle Uncle Harry never came to my bed during the night. If he was going to abuse me it would be before he went to bed. My mother normally went to bed about nine thirty p.m. and I was in bed by nine p.m. after I had finished my chores, washing up Uncle Harry's supper dishes and cleaning his and my brother's shoes. Once I was in bed I was told to turn my body away from the T.V. I knew that I had to keep my head down, and pretend that I was sleeping, even if I wasn't.

I am back there. I feel a coldness inside as I tell Helle about the oral abuse, which normally happens before Uncle Harry goes to bed. I can't tell Helle any details. I move on in my mind as if time has passed without me being conscious of the fact. I describe how scared I feel when I wake up in the middle of the night and I can see shapes, big dark shapes of 'Him' Uncle Harry. "He is watching me all through the night. He can see me at all times." I feel rigid with fear, unable to talk.

Helle and I talk about the images that I saw during the night I realised that the shapes that I saw were his work clothes and overcoat that he hung from the picture rail. He left them there over night ready to wear the next morning. He also told me that he was watching me. His clothes hanging there were a reminder.

Helle and I discuss my experiences of running away from home, the psychiatric hospitals and the Henderson. She begins to encourage me to seek advancement in my working life and I now take more of an active role in my children's schooling.

My first job, apart from my cleaning job, is as a youth worker. I work for two evenings a week and some Saturdays. I also continue with my cleaning job. I become very aware that my lack of reading and writing skills are a huge hindrance. Helle suggests that I attend an adult literacy class. I go along and join the class. It is made up of a small group of people and a teacher who is very bubbly and keen. I try to learn and feel such a sense of failure when I can't keep up. "What did the teacher mean when she talked about verbs, nouns and adjectives?" I just want to learn how to spell and read.

I say to Helle, "What if a new kid joins the youth club, I have to write down his name and I can't spell?"

Helle reassures me saying, "Ask him or her to spell it for you. Names are not always spelt the same way." Every time that I go into work at the youth centre I feel terrified that I am going to be seen as a thicko, stupid and completely unworthy. I like working with people, so I continue to work there and struggle with my reading and writing skills. After six months of working as a youth worker, I leave youth work and my morning cleaning job.

I have applied for a job at Islington Social Services at an adult social training day centre for people with learning difficulties. The Job is working as a kitchen assistant. The manager of the day centre knows my background and wants to help. She does help me by offering me an opportunity to prove myself.

I work from nine a.m. to one thirty p.m. in the kitchen helping the cook to make the morning tea, coffee and a midday meal for the clients and staff. After one thirty p.m., I go into various groups, as a volunteer, and work alongside a member of staff, teaching, encouraging and enabling clients to learn skills that will help them to become a little more independent. After six months I am promoted to care assistant. I start to see that I am a little more intelligent than I have given myself credit for. I can also see that my poor reading and writing skills will hold me back, although they have improved with my continued attendance at the adult literacy classes.

Helle says that she thinks that I need the specialised services of a dyslexic unit. There is a dyslexic unit at Guy's hospital. She refers me there and after an initial assessment I am offered two evening appointments a week.

I am receiving a lot of encouragement at work and at the dyslexic unit to develop my growing interest in the problems of people with learning disability. My newfound pleasure in learning sets me exploring different concepts.

I am learning about this new world that I have found. Helle is still holding me. I am seeing her twice a week for therapy and phoning her at weekends. A neighbour, who also works at Smithfield meat market with Uncle Harry, tells me that Uncle Harry has cancer and is dying. I phone my mother and make arrangements to go and visit.

I feel numb as I walk along the balcony and knock on the front door of the flat where I was brought up. I feel as if I am visiting the chamber of horrors. As I step inside the flat it seems much smaller than I remember. What used to be my brothers' bedroom has now become my mother and Uncle Harry's bedroom. My mother points for me to go into the sitting room. Memories of sitting in the corner, the put-u-up bed and Uncle Harry talking at me for hours came flooding back, although all the shabby furniture has been replaced with a new green suite, dining room table and chairs and a new dark green carpet.

My mother looks drawn. She tells me that she is managing and that Joe and Dennis are helping her. Dennis drives Uncle Harry to all his hospital appointments. She then goes on to tell me that the cancer has spread all over his body and that he is in terrible pain. She says, "I have just had the doctor around because he had a bad night. The doctor told me that he doesn't know how he is continuing to survive and that he can die at any time."

My mother led the way into their bedroom. I sit on a chair next to his bed. I am surprised because he is as fat as ever. I was expecting him to have lost a lot of weight. He asks me in a stern voice, "What have you got to say for yourself?"

I feel like a young child again who has been naughty. I tell him in an adult voice, "I have heard from your workmate about your illness." I go on to tell him, "I am working at a day centre as a Care Assistant I am enjoying working with the people there very much."

To my surprise he says, "I know about you working there. I know about everything, everything that you think or that you do. I'm watching you and I can see everything you do. I know that you go on swimming trips with the children and you shop in the Holloway Road."

A cold fear, the same fear that I felt when I was a child, sweeps over me.

I say, "I have to get back for the children now" and I head for the front door.

As I am leaving my mother says, "You know that this is your fault, don't you?"

I look at her. I am puzzled, I don't understand. "This is about you telling them about what happened."

I leave feeling dizzy and confused, so confused.

I tell Helle about what had happened. Helle says, "Pam, I think they are so hurtful to you and they always dump so much on to you that you ought to stay away from them, for your own sanity."

I never see Uncle Harry or my mother again. I heard about nine months later that he died in a hospice.

A few weeks after my visit to my mother and Uncle Harry, my brother Joe turns up at my house unannounced. Simon and the children are out. They are visiting Simon's parents. I notice that Joe has put on a lot of weight. He says that he has to come and see me because he has to tell me about how bad he is. He tells me how all men are bad to women and that he isn't to be trusted. He says, "Do you know that when we were in the children's home I was sexually abused by a member of staff? It wasn't just you."

Joe goes on to tell me how his doctor has sorted out a mental health group for him to attend. He continues to tell me with a smile and with great pride, "I went to their stupid group and I caused complete chaos, I wound them up, stupid bastards, if they think they are going to get me then they can think again."

I again feel as I did when I was a child: Joe talks and I listen, only this time I don't know what to say to him and I find him strange. He says, "Uncle Harry was mugged on the bus as he went to work one morning. Five youths jumped him and beat him up at five a.m. when he wasn't expecting it. The cancer came on about three months later. Stupid bastard, he should have been watching out."

Joe recalls how Uncle Harry tormented him when he was a child, "Do you remember, Pam, when he used to whisper 'Billy, Billy where are you?' Fucking bastard. He went on and on until I wanted to fucking knife him."

Billy is our father's name and Uncle Harry knew how to bait Joe. As Joe is talking my mind goes back to another occasion when Uncle Harry wound Joe up. He whispers, "Billy, Billy I know you're there Billy." Joe, who must have been a strong seventeen old, runs up behind Uncle Harry and smashes him across the back with one of the dining room chairs. All hell breaks lose. Nanny Donnelly, who was staying with us, ushers Joe out of the house and on to the balcony. My mother is screaming and Uncle Harry has picked himself up off the floor and is lunging at Joe. Joe runs off and I don't see him for days.

Joe's voice comes back into focus. He is saying, "Mum has retired from work early to look after Uncle Harry."

Joe looks at me and says, "I know I was bad and did bad things when we were growing up."

Joe then says, "Pam, I can't see you anymore because I have mixed feelings about you and I can't cope with what happened back then."

Joe leaves. I feel numb, sad and confused. I shall never see Joe again.
I tell Helle in my next session. I can't take it in. Joe, my brother who protected me, the one I admired and loved, tells me that he doesn't want to see me anymore.

I am still working at the day centre and for the first time in my life, apart from having Jay and Beth, I feel that what I am doing is worthwhile and I feel wanted. I am working with people who are needy, much needier than me. I know what it feels like to try and communicate and not be understood. I know what it feels like to be seen as different and not as valuable as the rest of the community. I find that I have a particular skill in communicating with profoundly disabled clients who are unable to communicate verbally. I am able to observe very closely and pick up subtle body language, which can indicate distress or the wishes of the client. I develop good relationships with the other members of staff at the day centre. I apply for and through a competitive interview I get the job of care officer. There are two posts, one at the day centre where I am working and one at another day centre in the borough. I am offered the choice. I am suitable for either post. I am well chuffed. I stay at the day centre where I have been working for the last eighteen months.
I feel such pride in my achievement. I am feeling very happy. My role at the day centre is to promote and develop sporting activities. I take groups of clients swimming and to the local leisure centres. I meet up with other staff from different day centres at the leisure centre and we organise our clients into teams to play basketball, table tennis or football together. Sometimes groups of clients from outside of the borough join us and teams compete against each other. This gives some of the clients an opportunity to mix with other people in their community.

I am very pleased when I become a swimming instructor and I become a qualified lifeguard. I liase with the local boys' school for clients from the day centre to use the school's swimming pool twice a week. This enables some of the more physically disabled clients to get out of the day centre and to go swimming once a week. I enjoy my work and I enjoy the people I work with. Work colleagues become friends, and we socialise together.

Most Friday evenings we stay on at work or go to each other's houses and in the summer we go to the pub and sit outside in the pub garden. Simon, Jay and Beth normally come with me. Christine, the day centre manager, drives to the school and collects my two children and her own little girl, who is the same age as Beth. During the school holidays Beth and Jay can come to work with me, although my holiday usually coincides with the school holidays.

As a family we spend Christmas day at Christine's house with her partner and her little girl. I have a group of friends that I can talk to. I am able to talk to them about almost anything, work issues, problems with my kids, lots of other issues and things we have in common. The problems that I had when I was a child and the entire childlike feelings that are evoked by my memories are kept for my sessions with Helle.

I apply to be seconded onto a social work course, The Certificate in Social Services. I don't know whether I will be accepted. Although my English and grammar have improved, I am still not able to write at an academic level. Most of my colleagues are graduates with a degree of one sort or another. Despite this, I work side by side with them and they never make me feel less than them. I go first for an interview with the assistant director of social services. He has known me since I was a client at the mental health day centre. When he has given his approval I am interviewed at Havering College. I just manage to scrape through the entrance exam and I am given a place on the C.S.S. course at Havering College.

I start my course in September 1984. I am at college two days a week. The borough provides extra study support for me. I see my study supervisor Felicity twice a week. She goes through my English and grammar with me. She also challenges my attitudes, ideas and concepts when necessary. I am challenged and supported and my communication skills develop in leaps and bounds.

The CSS course presents a different experience of 'teachers' from the one that I have previously had. I am expected to produce five assignments a term. I have to work hard at my written work; writing in an academic style doesn't come easily to me. Learning how to study, using a library and being able to talk in seminars are also new to me.

Whilst I am on the CSS course I am introduced to Rogerian counselling. I find it fascinating. I enjoy learning and practicing counselling skills, reading about counselling and using my newly learned skills as a worker. I pass the module with ease and am told, when my practice is observed, that the way I relate to my client is insightful, respectful and empathic.

I also learn about group work. One of my favourite assignments is observing and writing up a series of written process recordings on the weekly staff meeting explaining the dynamics of the group and my interpretation of what is happening. I learn and begin to understand group dynamics. Through reading and studying I start to become more aware of what is happening in the world, I develop a politically awareness and I have opinions on a range of different subjects. It is all very new to me that my opinions are of any interest.

On the CSS course, I make new friends and have a different experience of learning. At times it feels as if I am reliving my youth, in a positive way, rather than the destructive adolescence that I had experienced. It is only on a few occasions that my past affects my learning.

While taking part in an experiential exercise in working with adolescents, we are asked to get into groups of five and to think back to when we were teenagers and discus what issues were important to us at that time. To my amazement the other students are talking about having spots, not enough pocket money and having arguments with their parents about what time they had to be home from a party, or not having done their homework. I can't relate to this and I panic. I feel sick as my head spins and I half go back into the past. I know that it is not appropriate to share my experiences and I manage to sit with my confusion and panic. My panicky feelings subside and I feel very different from the other students. I feel as if I have come from another planet and that I have no right to be here. I do not belong. I am here under false pretences. I feel as if they are going to catch me out and send me away.

My educational experiences are feeding back into my therapy sessions with Helle. Helle helps me to talk things through, and to work through any difficult feelings.

I frequently join my colleagues and friends on peace demonstrations at Greenham. On one occasion demonstrators are asked to observe a period of silence. My friends and I decide to communicate in Makaton, a form of sign language used when working with learning disabled clients. Just for this moment I feel as if I belong with this group of people. I understand what they are about and my world opens up with all sorts of possibilities that I had no knowledge of just five or six years ago.

Christine, my manager and friend, who works with me at the day centre has a new partner, who is part of the A.N.C.. He has managed to get out of South Africa before being arrested. Christine and her partner tell Simon and me about what is happening in South Africa. We are introduced to lots of their friends who are involved in the A.N.C. We go with Christine to a fund raising concert. A group of black South African singers perform on stage, their music is moving and it puts me in touch with their struggle. I hear some weeks after seeing this performance that one of the leading singers was shot dead when she returned to South Africa. It is something that makes me feel very close to the situation, when I had witnessed such a vibrant, wonderful singer, and she has been shot dead for nothing more than her skin colour, her struggle against injustice and for speaking out for something that she believed in.

When I pass the CSS course Christine and Felicity tell me how proud the training section and the assistant director are of my achievement in passing the course. A couple of months after finishing my course I decide to move from the day centre and work in a residential setting. My thinking is that this move will give me more experience and I will be able to apply for promotion. The day centre holds a leaving party for me and for passing my course. A large number of people, who work in the borough, have come to my party, and this overwhelms me.
Certain people have taken a big risk with me, firstly by giving me my first job and then supporting me through the various stages of my career and I feel very grateful to those people for giving me such a chance.

Jay and Beth are in secondary school. Beth spends her time with friends who are children from middle class families. A few of these children have well-known parents and relatives and I think they send their children to a state school because of their socialist beliefs. Jay insists on remaining with his working class roots. His friends are the boys who live on the estate where we live. He often says to me, "Mum why can't you just be ordinary like the other kid's mums? Why are you always studying and so political?"

The truth was I didn't feel that I really belonged in either group. When Beth is going away with her friend's family I am aware that her friend has a famous socialist aunty and her friend's mother is a well-known illustrator of children's books. On other occasions Beth stays over night with another one of her friends whose father is a famous barrister. I have to go to her friend's houses and talk to their parents to find out what arrangements have been made and sometimes to collect Beth when she needs to come home. Simon now leaves this sort of thing to me, I feel out of my depth and I know that I can't reciprocate. I may have similar political beliefs to these parents, but I don't have their education or money and neither does Beth. Equally, when Jay goes on holiday to Ireland with his friend's family who live on our estate, I feel different. I know that I am known as the weirdo with left wing ideas and a history of mental illness. Again I don't feel that I fit in with this group of people.

I am doing well. I am growing and learning. Simon, however, becomes one of Maggie Thatcher's victims. He is made redundant from the firm where he has worked for the past ten years and at thirty-five is finding it difficult to find another job. For some months Simon stays at home and keeps house while I go out to work. Friends of ours and I try to persuade Simon to go back to college, to become a mature student and acquire skills in a different line of work. He is very good at languages and can already speak French and German, so we think that he can develop these languages as well as learning others and perhaps become a linguist. He refuses.

Simon becomes ill. He is taken into hospital and has an operation to remove a kidney stone. He takes a few weeks to recover. He tells me, "The doctors told me that I almost died whilst I was in surgery." He is also told that he has to go back into hospital to have part of his parathyroid gland removed as this organ is causing too much calcium to be produced, which may cause further kidney stones to develop. I visit Simon every day in hospital and I am very worried about him. He isn't his normal self. When the children and I visit, he doesn't seem to want us there and when Simon comes out of hospital, he is depressed and he spends a lot of time on his own sitting in the living room with his head phones on, listening to music.

Helle thinks that it is time for my therapy with her to come to an end. She says, "Perhaps we can become colleagues rather than therapist and client."

I don't know that I am ready to stop my therapy with Helle. I think that I am going to need some persuading.

We decide to write an article together, which is published in the 'British Journal of Psychotherapy 1986'. Helle suggests and introduces me to an organisation that she belongs to called 'Workshops In Living and Learning' (WILL London). The group is made up of psychotherapists from The London Centre for Psychotherapists and other people who are involved in working with people.

We work in groups using themes as a way of communicating ideas and feelings. Members of the group do not make interpretations on what another member of the group is talking about. They simply make their contribution by stating their own experiences, ideas and feelings. For example, the theme might be "Working with Teenagers". This is broken down into sub themes e.g. Think about a situation that brought you into contact with teenagers, this might be with your own children, or teenagers with whom you work. You might want to talk about your own experiences of being a teenager. Then whoever has something to say on the subject will start the discussion.

Members run groups for social services staff and for members of the public. There are a few occasions when I am involved in the running of groups with a more experienced member of WILL London.

For my friends and family, deciding on a date for finishing my therapy with Helle and my working towards that date seems very straightforward. For me it is hell. I plead with her, "You can't do this to me. I'm not ready and I don't know how I will manage without you."

It feels like she is killing a part of me off. Helle says, "We must work towards finishing, Pam. I am beginning to feel very tired, and it is time for you to move on. When you come into my consulting room, I want you to sit in a chair, not to lie on the couch."

I sit with my head down, the room is spinning and I hate her. She is just someone else who has let me down. Helle says, "Why don't you stop sulking? Go out of the room and come back in, and start again."

This is too much. I kick her table over and walk out, only to return half an hour later saying that I am sorry and that I will try, but I have to lie down. I can't sit facing her. That will be too much. To sit and face her would mean looking at her and although I can do this at WILL London, I cannot do it in her consulting room.

Helle agrees to let me lie on the couch for my sessions with her. She tries to get me to look at her but I can't, not in this place. There are times at WILL London when my envy and rage goes into overdrive. These are times when Helle talks about her family or she offers to give one of the other members of the group a lift in her car. We talk about the envy and the rage in my therapy sessions.

Nine months has passed since I started working at the residential hostel for people with learning disabilities. A new project is being advertised within Islington Social Services, a joint funded project with the health service, although the staff are to be employed by social services. The job involves working with adults with learning disabilities, who are in long stay hospitals and are returning to their borough of origin. The staff will manage the clients' day care needs as well as supporting them to live in their own homes. I apply for the deputy manager's post, and I am successful. The interview panel is unable to appoint a manager at this time and I become the acting manager.

The work that is involved is completely new to me. It is my responsibility to lead a team of ten staff, to select eight people with learning disabilities from various long stay hospitals and to resettle them in Islington where they originated. We are based in an old building, while the day centre, which will be our permanent base, is refurbished. The two houses that have been converted into four two-bedroom flats, didn't initially meet the health and safety standards for staff to be able to work there. This means that the team and I have to visit and work with the clients at the long stay hospitals until the refurbishment is finished.

When I first visit Harperbury Hospital, I think that I have been transported back in time. The huge palatial grounds remind me of the children's home. The song, " The Teddy bear's picnic" comes into my mind. Panic engulfs me. I have to push it away.
I also go to St Lawrence's Hospital and learn that most of the patients there have been there since they were young adolescents, and are now in their fifties. This really upsets

me. I also think what a lucky escape I had when I was in the psychiatric hospital and it was recommended that I be sent to a special hospital. I am still grateful to the magistrate who said no to that recommendation.

I am working with one of my old colleagues, Claire B, who I know from the day centre. She also joins WILL London with me. We know each other well and Claire is a great support to me in my working life. I am finding this job upsetting and stressful, at times.

It is coming close to the date that Helle and I have agreed to finish therapy. I am functioning at work and for the most part at home, although there is a part of me that I have switched off. I am now resigned to the fact that therapy is going to finish and the child part of me has to be managed by myself. The only way that I know how to do this is to split her off from my functioning adult. I often feel as if I have switched on to automatic pilot when childlike feelings surface.

Simon has found himself a temporary job, which he hopes will become permanent at some point. It is not very well paid but it is better than having no job at all.

He starts to become secretive and insists on going out on his own on in the evenings after work. I ask him, "Where are you going?"

He angrily replies, "Mind your own business. I don't have to tell you anything."

I find out, after being away for three days attending a conference for my work, that Simon has spent one of the nights away from home. Beth tells me, "I was scared when you were away, mum. I was scared because Dad didn't come home one night."

Simon, who should have been at home looking after both Beth and Jay, hadn't returned until early the next morning after going out for the evening.

I wait until Beth has gone out to her friend's house, then I confront Simon, "How could you leave the kids alone all night? They are only fifteen and sixteen years old."

He says very calmly, "I have met someone else. I'm planning to leave home when Beth reaches the age of sixteen. I don't love you, I never have, but I always told myself that I would stay until the children had reached sixteen."

I am stunned. Where did this magical age of sixteen fit in? I feel numb and meekly agree that he can stay until he decides when to leave. I carry on working and I come home and act as if everything is normal. Simon carries on working. He goes out most evenings, returning home in the early hours of the morning. After two weeks it all comes to a head. Simon stays out all night on Saturday night. I phone the police station and the local hospitals because I am afraid that he has had an accident.

Simon returns home at midday on Sunday. I ask him, "Where have you been? I have been going out of my mind with worry."

He says, "You shouldn't have worried about me. I have had a great time with one of the women from work."

He begins to tell me about her, "She is nineteen. I met her at work and I have fallen in love with her. Do you know that when she was a child she had also been sexually abused? A stranger abused her. It's sad. She has just lost her father, so she needs me at the moment. You can understand that, can't you?"

I walk out of the house. I have to get some air, I can't take in all of this. He is like a teenager who is asking for his mother's approval. I go back home and find that he has gone out to the pub. I find myself packing his case. As I am packing a rage sets in. I rip his shirts to shreds and stuff them in the case. When he returns from the pub, before he can get inside the front door, I throw his case at him and tell him to piss off.

He has the nerve to tell me that he can't leave today because she, his girl friend is away visiting her mother. That makes me even angrier. I slam the door in his face.

I have to explain to Jay and Beth what has happened. They were both out with their friends when their dad and I were arguing. Beth wants to see her dad. Jay remains quiet.

I don't hear from Simon for two weeks. I arrive home from work to find him slumped in a chair with his headphones on. I have picked up some vegetables for the evening meal. Simon takes off his headphones, looks at the carrier bag that I am holding and says, "You shouldn't shop there. You should shop at the other greengrocers; they have better and cheaper veg."

He goes on to tell me that Beth is in her room and that she has gone there after he told her that she shouldn't sit with her shoes on the furniture.

This is weird. I can't make sense of what this man is saying. I think that he has lost the plot. I remind him, "Simon, you have left home. It's no longer any of your damn business where I shop or whether Beth puts her shoes on the furniture."

I also tell him that both Beth and Jay want to spend some time with him. He says that he doesn't feel that he can cope with that at the moment but gives me a number where they can contact him. Simon leaves. I can't believe what has happened. We have known each other for eighteen years and it is over within two weeks.

Jay arrives home saying that he has packed in his job. He is an apprentice printer. I ask him, "What do you think you are doing? If you are not going to work then you need to go back to school."

He refuses. Beth starts to come home late, telling me that it is none of my business about where she has been or what she is doing. I think that I am losing control. Everything is going haywire. I ask the children to come to family therapy with me. I have worked it out with Helle and Pat, my friend, that the situation with Joe and Beth's father leaving, might have reminded the youngsters of my breakdown and the time when they went into care. What they need is for me to hold myself together for them. Jay and Beth attend the first appointment at the Tavistock Clinic with me, only to say that it is a waste of time and there is nothing to talk about.

I feel as if I am on a roller-coaster, everything is moving so fast, I don't have time to digest what has just happened before the next thing comes and hits me in the face.

My manager arrives at my place of work on Monday morning. We don't have a meeting arranged and I am perplexed as to why he is here. Mark says, "Pam, I am concerned about your daughter Beth. Did you know that she went to see a social worker near to your home last week? Beth told Glen, the social worker, that she wants to leave home."

Beth has just turned fifteen and Glen knows me. He has discreetly let Mark know that Beth has been to see him.

I explain to Mark what has been happening at home. Mark is very supportive. He explains that there is a case file about my children and myself on record and that he is going to ask the Assistant Director to put a stop on any social worker having access to it without going through the Assistant Director first. He also arranges to have separate supervision slots with me that are not about work issues. He hopes that this will enable me to work out strategies to cope with Beth and Jay.

Meanwhile I continue to work with Helle on trying to understand and come to terms with the sudden breakdown of my marriage. I ask, "Why hadn't I seen it coming? I knew that Simon was depressed and that he had lost his job."

The way that I make sense of it in the end is to acknowledge that Simon has for the most part of our relationship been the stronger one who has propped me up. Others have seen me as the weak un-together wife who has to be supported by her strong husband. The roles have changed. I am now an independent, educated woman who earns a good income whilst Simon has been unemployed and now has taken work that has less pay and status. I no longer need Simon in quite the same way and I think that he cannot cope with the role reversal. The reason for his attraction to another woman is that our sexual relationship has never been as close or as passionate as Simon would have liked. Too much damage has been done to the sexual side of me.

I am at a large area meeting. The meeting is taking place at my place of work. After the meeting, the Assistant Director calls me to one side and tells me that my daughter was causing a commotion at head office on the Friday evening. "She had demanded to see someone who could help her to leave home." The Assistant Director went on to say, "Beth refused to leave the building until she was seen, and when I went to see her, Beth told me that she has a black boyfriend and her mother is a racist,", a comment that would be certain to get her attention. I feel exasperated by Beth's behaviour. I apologise to the Assistant Director on Beth's behalf and say that I will talk to Beth.

When I get home I try to talk to Beth about her behaviour and what she had said. Beth flounces into her room saying, "I don't have to talk about anything and I'm leaving home."

I attempt to reason with her, as on other occasions, but I get nowhere. Jay who is still refusing to work tells me that it is my fault that his father has left. He says, "If you had stayed a cleaner, Mum, it would have been O.K. Dad wouldn't have left us." I think that their father leaving in the way that he did and the fact that he doesn't have much contact with them is having a profound effect on both of them.

I feel that I am being severely punished by my children. Simon who hasn't been near or by is safely out of their reach.

Beth leaves home. She leaves a note to say that she is staying at a friend's squat. She also leaves me the address of where she is staying. When I meet with my work manager, Mark, we work out a strategy whereby I will visit Beth at the squat and tell her that I need to make sure that she is O.K. and I will also make it very clear that when she wants to come home my door will be open to her. When I go to visit Beth I find it so difficult to remain calm about her being in this smelly unsafe place. I want to pick her up and take her home. I don't. I follow the strategy that Mark and I have discussed. Within two days Beth is safely back home and back at school.

When Jay reaches seventeen, he decides to go abroad to find work. He stays in the Canary Islands working for six months.

On his return he is still unsettled and we have numerous arguments about his behaviour and his general attitude towards me. Jay moves in with a girlfriend and leaves home. Our relationship remains unsettled.

Some time later Jay travels to Africa as a volunteer working abroad. He tells me that this experience has changed the way he views the world and his situation. He has experienced people who have nothing and yet who can be so generous. I start to have and continue to have a good relationship with both Jay and Beth.

I know that my therapy with Helle is drawing to a close. With all that is going on, there is no time or space for me to work through ending my therapy with Helle. It is necessary for me to be there for Jay and Beth. There are times when I get home from work that the only way that I can relax and stop the pain inside is to drink a couple of cans of beer or a few glasses of wine. I start to break my own rules about only having a drink at weekends.

I start to develop problems with walking, my legs seem to seize up or they simply collapse on me. I go to the gym twice a week thinking that exercise might help but my back starts to hurt me and I find walking almost impossible. I have to take time off work and I go to see an osteopath. She says that whenever she approaches me to treat my back, my whole body tenses up as if I am going to be hit. She also thinks that the length of my bones seem too short for the length of the muscles, so I appear to have very over developed muscles, much the same as appears in dwarfism but not to the same extent. She treats my back for a slipped disc over a period of several months.

In 1989 Helle suggests that I leave therapy and I am not to contact her or see her for six to eight months. If I can manage this, then we can go on holiday together. The plan is that we visit India. When I leave therapy I feel numb and over the weeks my drinking increases, although I can still go to work and function. The crying child inside me comes and goes and I know that I have to shut it up, otherwise the sadness and rage will take me over and then I will be in trouble.
Friends and my osteopath are there for me. Whenever I am quiet and withdrawn and I drink too much, they don't seem to judge me. They just accept that I am going through a difficult time.

Anna, one of my friends who I work with, is gay and she starts to ask me about my sexuality. She says, "I have noticed that since you have broken up with Simon you haven't shown any interest in other men and all of your friends are female."

I think to myself: she is right, the most intimate relationships that I have had for most of my life have been with women, the only boys or men that I ever had love feelings for are my son and my brother Joe. I don't know whether this means that I am gay, I have never slept with a woman or had any sort of romantic relationship with another woman. I agree to go to a lesbian club with Anna. I start to question my sexuality.

Beth has met a young man, she is out of the house with him or working and I don't see much of her. Jay has moved out to his own council flat on Brecknock Road.

Helle phones me. She tells me that she really isn't very well and that if we are going to make our trip together it needs to be now. I make arrangements to see her at the London Centre for Psychotherapy on the following Tuesday.

REFLECTIONS
Chapter Seven

Some matters were not as straightforward chronologically as the account may seem to indicate. I stayed for a long time at the infant stage, in therapy, but took time to get there in the first place. Later on, my regression in therapy varied from session to session and even within sessions. Helle's skill at disentangling "How old are you now?"

helped me to make sense of my history, and link my feelings with the scraps of information that I had from my mother and nanny Donnelly.

I never saw my brother Joe from the time when he visited to this day but I did read in the newspaper that his now grown up daughter had chronic mental health problems and heard on the grapevine that his sons had entered into the world of criminality.

Referring to my working life, I think that there was much more emphasis on helping people like me to achieve in those days. The emphasis was on working with and caring about people. The individuals who entered the social work profession had very strong beliefs that the job was more than just earning a living. They truly cared about people and social injustice. It was a particular growth time in social concern and social work was highly regarded. A lot of resources went into training and development of staff, which enabled the staff to work as a team. During the Thatcher era the ethos changed and became less caring of those who were less fortunate or less able in society. It went back to the ideas prevalent in my childhood, selecting out the deserving and the undeserving. It remains like this today. Today it would not be possible for me to achieve as I did. I would not have been given the opportunity.

Budgets and the cost of provision becomes more important than the quality of care given to the client. This had a knock on effect on the staff in that they were less supported. There was much more emphasis on getting volunteers to do the work of trained professionals and a lot of work went over to private and voluntary services. The Thatcher era and its "Get on your bike" attitudes changed the moral and ethical views of the nation resulting in a much harder society in which people were only out for themselves and their own advantage.

CHAPTER EIGHT
FAREWELL TO HELLE

I meet with Helle as arranged at L.C.P. I walk into her consulting room and I feel concerned. She looks so tired and she has already told me that she hasn't been well. She tells me, "I have been for tests at the hospital, Pam, and although I think that everything is going to be all right, I need to be cautious about where we go on holiday, I need to have medical facilities nearby in case I need them. I think that travelling to India will be rather risky. Have you any ideas about where else you might like us to go on holiday?"
I couldn't really think of anywhere. It feels strange being here in Helle's consulting room and talking to her about holidays. I am also preoccupied with my thoughts about her health. I am worried and I want to ask her more about what is happening with her but feel that I shouldn't probe. Helle suggests going to Israel and it feels like a good choice. I leave after having made arrangements to meet Helle at Camden Town where we can book our holiday with a travel agent that I have used before.

I go home and I think about Israel being a good choice, I think about my mother and my mother's family. From the information that my mother gave me and from what I remember as a child, my mother came from a Jewish family, her maiden name was Samuels, my grandmother was a businesswoman in the world of fashion and, before the Second World War, she travelled to Paris frequently in connection with her business. My mother apparently came from a well to do, middle class, non-practicing Jewish family. She was the twelfth child to be born into a family of fourteen children and it seemed that the last three children, her sister, brother and herself were more or less brought up by her older sisters and brothers.

My mother didn't tell me much about her father, except that he was a quiet, self-contained man whom she didn't know that well. Both of my mother's parents had been disowned by their families for marrying against their parents' wishes.

My mother always seemed to me to be a nervous woman who needed a man to look after her. From what I saw of my mother's older brothers and sisters, they didn't seem to need to be looked after, although my mother's sister Joan did marry a man twenty years her senior and aunty Vi was a nervous, gentle woman and married to a very mild mannered man.

Uncle Harry always ridiculed aunty Vi and her husband, who always seemed to have colds when we saw them. He said as he laughed, "Mr Sniff and Mrs Snuff, the fucking weaklings, are visiting today."

Most of my mother's family stayed away from Uncle Harry. My mother said this was due to the fact that my grandmother left money in her will to my mother's older brother and sister, and they sold my grandmother's land. Uncle Harry's resentment and envy came out in ridicule of my mother's Jewish mannerisms. He also ridiculed her family and said they were like all Jews, tight with their money. According to Uncle Harry, my mother's brothers and sisters already had enough money, whereas my mother had very little. From what I remember of my mother's family, they did live in big houses, except for Aunty Rachel, who lived in a flat off Upper Street. I remember, when I was about seven or eight, my mother taking me to her older brother's house in Brownswood Road, and I think that it was the same house that my grandmother lived in when she was alive. There was a smell of matzo biscuits. I smelt the same smell many years later when I went inside a Jewish household in Lordship Lane. I remembered it with pleasure. Uncle Bert was always happy and joking, his wife was warm and friendly.

In April 1990 Helle and I met at Heathrow Airport, ready to fly off to Israel. Jay and Beth came to the airport with me. It is the first time that Jay and Beth meet Helle and there is time for a cup of coffee and chat together, before Helle and I go through passport control. We arrive at Tel-Aviv airport, collect the hire car and Helle drives us to a small hotel, which is situated on the sea front. Helle takes a rest in her room before we meet in the hotel lobby to go for lunch. We have lunch at a small bistro, where I eat French onion soup for the first time. After lunch we go for a short walk along the front before settling on the beach against some rocks, which provide some shade. Almost as soon as we are settled, Helle looks at me. She looks worried. She says, "Pam, I need to tell you that I am very ill."

I am nervous about what she is going to tell me. Helle continues, "When I was in my forties I had stomach cancer. I had a lot of radiotherapy, which has damaged my skin. Due to the amount of radiotherapy that I had, the doctors are unable to operate on me to check whether the stomach cancer has returned. Pam, I know that I have cancer and I don't have long to live. This is why we had to take our holiday sooner than planned."

I sit listening to Helle's words. I feel stunned. My face must go white because Helle asks me if I am O.K. and says, "It's all right to cry, crying helps us to cleanse away the pain."

This is something that Helle has said to me many times in therapy, but I can never manage to cry even if it feels as if I am crying inside. I can't cry now either, I just feel numb, shocked and so sad. This is terrible news that I don't want to be true.

We wander back to our hotel because Helle feels exhausted and thinks she is going to be sick. We stay in Tel-Aviv the following day, spending most of the day on the beach. Helle tells me more about her illness and her life. I discover that she has three grown up children, a girl and two boys. She says, "I married a Scotsman and we live in

Epsom. My father was a doctor and during the war, when Denmark was occupied, my family were involved with the resistance movement. My father being the local G.P. in the village where we lived meant that he was a man with influence and he was a central figure in the resistance movement. I used to run messages on my bike for my father to other resistance members."

I remember when in the early part of my therapy with Helle I got very upset because she was going on holiday for a month. She gave me her Star of David, which hung around her neck, as a keepsake for whist she was away. During the war when the Nazis ordered all Jews to wear the Star of David the King of Denmark came out wearing a Star of David and the Danish people followed him in this. She told me at the time that she gave it to me that she wears it as a reminder that such an atrocity should never be allowed to happen again. The Star of David has a huge meaning for her. Here I am in Israel still wearing her Star of David. I feel very proud to know this woman and to be a part of her life.

I talk to Helle about having thoughts about my sexuality. Helle finds this difficult and says, "Pam, if you are a lesbian then I will feel that myself and the therapy are partly responsible."

"I can't make that out. I don't understand how you can be responsible," I say.

Helle says, "Maybe I allowed you too much time in the regression stage of your therapy and this has somehow damaged your sexuality."

"No, Helle, I disagree with you. The love feelings that I felt in the regressive stage are childlike and different. Wanting to have a relationship with a woman is very different to what I felt for you."

I also talk to Helle about starting a counselling course in September. The one that I am interested in is called The Pellin Institute. It is quite a popular course with my female friends and although the course is open to both sexes it is mostly women that apply for and go on to it. Helle is keen for me to sign up for a group therapy course that is running at Goldsmiths. We talk about the pros and cons of both courses and she tells me that she will be happy with whichever course I choose. Helle still feels like mum to me and I am glad to get her approval.

On the third day of our holiday we travel by hire car to Jerusalem, where we stay in a hostel. Helle is really sick in the evening. She has to go straight to her room and goes to bed early. I discover that Helle can't eat big meals and needs to eat little and often. She carries sachets of dried soup and mint leaves. She puts the mint leaves into hot water, which she says sooths her stomach. There are times when we go into a café and I feel a little embarrassed. Helle asks for two cups of hot water and says when asked, "No, thank you, I don't want anything else. Two cups of hot water will be fine."

Helle seems to need to eat something about every two to three hours and then whatever she has to eat or drink is rejected by her body half an hour later. She is violently sick and has diarrhoea. I am very worried about her. I also feel so nervous. I don't understand why I feel bereft as if I have been abandoned in this strange place to fend for myself when Helle has to take to her bed.

I have sleepless nights and I can't believe it when I see Helle the following morning. She has recovered and is eager to get on with what she has planned for the day.

We make our way to the inner city of Jerusalem. The weather is vile. It is April and it is raining hailstones and very cold. We spend most of the day looking in the different parts of the old city. There is the Jewish part, the Arab part and the Christian part. It soon becomes clear to me that I can't tell the difference between the Arabs and the Jewish people.

On the way back to the hostel where we are staying, Helle stops at a hotel outside the old city. She starts to talk to the man on reception. He is an Arab man. She asks him about the city and then goes on to ask him what he thinks of the troubles and what is happening in Israel and how he thinks a solution can be found. She also asks if it is safe for us to travel around unescorted. He says, "In my opinion, it is safe for two women to travel anywhere they want to in Israel without the fear of being attacked by Arab people. Arab men will not attack two women on their own."
I can't be paying attention and I must have gone somewhere else in my mind because I don't know how they have reached this part of their conversation.
Helle later points out how nervous I become when in the company of a strange man.

Helle has arranged for us to stay on a Kibbutz for a couple of nights. She drives us to a Kibbutz near Haifa. While we are staying on the Kibbutz, Helle has an appointment with a Rabbi, who is also a psychotherapist. While she is meeting with him I am shown around the outside of the Kibbutz. It is in a compound surrounded by a high-wired fence. Through the fence, I can see a wonderful, lush countryside. The young woman who is showing me around says they have the high-wired fence because Arabs have attacked them and they need to stay vigilant at all times.
After our evening meal, Helle and I chat to a woman, who is very interesting. She works with people who survived the holocaust and their families. She tells us that she has been in Israel since the end of the Second World War. She helped to set up the Kibbutz since she arrived in Israel from England. She goes on to explain that she was a German Jewish child who, together with her sister, had been sent to a family in Newcastle for the duration of the war. After the war was over, she discovered that her entire family had been killed. She never returned to Germany.

Both she and her sister settled in Israel. I am intrigued with her story. She reminds me of a nun. She is tall and slim with dark hair and eyes. She talks in a soft gentle way and there is an air of serenity about her. She tells us that she never married. "Survivors of the holocaust tended to marry other survivors. I think that the children of the survivors carry the unspeakable scars and the pain that their parents couldn't bear to speak of."

I feel humbled by this woman. She has suffered huge losses of her own and yet she devotes her life to looking after others.

Helle and I spend the next morning at the Sea of Galilee. It is springtime, the weather has brightened up and it all looks very beautiful. We drive back to the Kibbutz to spend our last night there. Helle gets into a conversation with a young man about his thoughts on the conflict between the Jewish settlers and the Arabs. The young man answers her politely. Helle becomes very provocative and the young man gets angry although the conversation goes back to being a harmonious one. I ask Helle, "Why did you make him so angry?"

She smiles and says, "I wanted to see how he really felt about what was happening."

We travel to Haifa and stay in a posh hotel. Helle says that this is her treat. Helle remains well and I feel so happy to be with her. I am finding out so much more about her and how she interacts with people. I look after her by carrying her bags and fetching her mint tea or soup. Helle isn't one for being looked after. She lets me do these things for her and she also lets me know that she is letting me look after her in this way.

We visit the Dead Sea. It is surrounded by desert. I manage to get a few photographs of Helle. She is always full of surprises and I am seeing a side to Helle that I have never experienced before. She is wearing a gilet, which she tells me she has brought from a jumble sale in Epsom, the area where she lives. She also wears a large full brimmed hat and baggy trousers. She tells me that she also brought these from a jumble sale. She makes me smile because she looks like an eccentric older woman.

I want to take photographs of different aspects of the desert. I thought that a desert would just look like a desert but it's like looking at any other landscape: you can get different views depending on at which angle you're pointing your camera. I am trying to get a snapshot which doesn't include telegraph poles. Helle asks me, "What are you trying to do, Pam?" I explain. She smiles and says, "But that's what is there. Why try to hide the telegraph poles when they are part of the landscape? It's like trying to hide parts of yourself, it isn't necessary."

While we are driving back to our hotel from our walk in the desert, Helle decides to veer off the main road and goes onto a much narrower road. We are driving for quite a while before we come to a small village. There are goats in the middle of the road and Helle has to drive very slowly in case our car hit one of the goats. Before we know it we are in the middle of the village. Women and children are standing outside their houses. They come towards the car and some of the older children start spitting at us. They are also shouting at us. I feel terrified but Helle calmly takes out her Danish flag from the glove compartment of the car and waves it out of her side window. She says to me without looking at me, "Smile and wave at them. Let them know that we are friendly. We will be O.K because I am flying the Danish flag." I smile and wave as she told me but I am thinking to myself we are driving a hired car with Israeli number plates and will children recognise the Danish flag?

We are only in that situation for ten minutes or so but it seems like ages and I am so relieved to be safe. Once we get past the village Helle continues to drive along this narrow road. Then, as the road turns, we can see an armed military vehicle coming towards us. It is the Israeli army. They ask us what we are doing here and want to see our passports and Helle's driving licence. Once they are satisfied that we aren't up to anything, they escort our car back onto the main highway, telling us that when we stray off the main road we are putting ourselves in grave danger.

Helle can't understand why I have got so frightened. She asks me, "Where is your sense of adventure?"
Helle talks about going to one of the Palestinian refugee camps. I do not want to go there but she only gives up the idea, much to my relief, when several different people tell her that she won't be allowed to enter a refugee camp.

We drive to Eilat for the day. Along the way we are stopped by the police for speeding. Helle is driving extremely fast. The policeman warns her that it is a dangerous road and she needs to take care. The speed that Helle was driving at has made me feel nervous. Helle says, "I thought you would enjoy that. When my children were younger they loved it when I drove fast."
I explain to Helle that, in fact, I am a person who even avoids fun fairs because I don't like the sensation of speed. We manage to reach Eilat and I swim amongst the most beautiful coral reef. On the way home Helle has to stop frequently to rest. I am aware that Helle has made this trip to the coast for me, even though driving such a distance has completely tired her out.

It's our last day and we are back in Jerusalem. The weather is better than it was the last time that we were here. It is a Saturday and we are invited into someone's house. The man whose house we are in explains that today is his son's wedding day and that it is a Jewish custom to invite strangers in and offer them a drink and some food. There are also other strangers who have been invited in. I ask about taking a photograph. I am told that I can take a photo but Jewish people can't because it is their Sabbath. Helle talks to our host for a good while asking about his faith and his customs, and then we thank him and leave.

We make our way back to the hostel where we were staying and pack. The hire car has to be back by midnight. We drive there in good time and go straight to the airport although our flight is not until six the following morning. We sit in the airport with our luggage. Then Helle sees a group of Arab people who are also waiting for a flight. Helle goes and sits with them and I follow her. She talks to them for about an hour before they go through passport control for their flight. We settle down for the night as we still have a long wait before checking in for our flight. Helle produces a thermal blanket. It looks like a space blanket. It is a thin silver piece of cloth. She wraps this blanket around herself and goes to sleep in a chair. I can't sleep. I feel that I need to keep awake in case something dangerous happens or our luggage gets stolen.

We go through passport control at five the following morning. We are both asked to step aside and are taken into two separate interview rooms. I am asked about our stay in Israel. Where have we been? Who did we see? Where did we go and on what dates? This type of questioning goes on for an hour or so. I am then taken into another room. Helle is there, she is protesting about her luggage being searched by airport security staff. At one point a security man takes out her camera and asks, "What is this?" Helle snatches the camera from him, opens up the camera case and points the camera at him saying, "Smile, smile for the camera."

I look at her and shake my head, indicating no, don't wind him up. Helle is furious with the officials. She says, "You ought to be ashamed of yourselves. The Nazis treated me like this when Denmark was occupied. I wasn't frightened then and I won't be intimidated now." With that we were escorted onto the plane. No duty free shopping on this trip!

Helle sleeps for most of the journey home. She looks tired and very unwell. I take this time to reflect on our holiday together. Although Helle says that she is not afraid to die, I think that she is very angry and I think that her anger exacerbates her normal rebellious nature although, to be fair, I had not voiced my fears perhaps because of a fear of rejection. Helle is in any case a risk-taker. She demonstrated this by agreeing to take me on for psychotherapy when so many other therapists had refused.

Helle's son meets her at the airport and they leave me very sharply with a quick wave. She says, "Bye, I will be in contact with you soon."

I suddenly feel very alone and frightened. Something inside me is crying as I make my way home on the tube. I don't hear from Helle for about six weeks although I have sent her copies of some of the photographs that I have taken.

Beth announces that she has fallen pregnant and I am worried about her because I don't think that her relationship with Andrew, her partner, will last.

I am plodding along with work and I join a lesbian organization that meets up one Saturday in three. Groups of women tend to socialise together after the Saturday afternoon meeting has finished and I join in with this.

Helle phones me and asks if I would like to visit her at her house, and we make arrangements for me to visit her at the weekend. I take the train to Epsom and Helle meets me at the station. She looks terrible. She has lost so much weight. She explains that she hasn't been in touch because, on her return from our trip, she had become so ill that she was taken into hospital. She says, "The hospital has done some tests, including a blood test, and has put a camera into my stomach to see what is happening but they are still none the wiser as to what is wrong with me. I shouldn't really be driving but I am determined to carry on as normally as possible."

We reach Helle's house and I notice that she has my photographs of the desert in Israel, which I have sent to her. She has enlarged them and has them hanging in her hallway. Helle continues to tell me about her illness. She is angry with the medics. She tells me of an incident when a young nurse called her 'dear'. Helle says, "I told her that I was not her 'dear', she hardly knew me." She was equally scathing about the doctors.

Helle is very ill and she is adamant that she is going to die. She insists that she has cancer and hates 'being an invalid'. She says, "I am not afraid of death and if it is time, then I am ready, but I will not be pulled about, patronised and told what to do." From this I gather she means that she has been told to stop smoking. Helle manages a small walk with me around her garden as I tell her about Beth's news.

I take a taxi back to the station, having arranged with Helle to visit again in two weeks time. I continue to visit Helle throughout the summer. I get to meet her husband and one of her sons. It is her son who meets me from the station and takes me back to the station when I am ready to go home. Helle and I talk about Beth's pregnancy. She asks me about Beth's fears and concerns and then advises me on how best to support her. Helle is also interested in Jay and what he is doing. I talk to her about my difficulties at work and how I manage a group of staff and the clients that I am responsible for. I often discuss and take advice from Helle as to how I can manage my conflicting feelings about certain polices that I am expected to carry out, regardless of whether I believe in them or not. As I talk with Helle, I feel like a young woman who is getting advice from an aunty or her mother and when it is time to leave Helle, I feel crying pains in my tummy and it takes me a day or two to get myself back together again.

As far as I understand, Helle continues to work at home and works from L.C.P. albeit for fewer hours. Helle continues to lose weight and now needs the aid of a walking stick to help her with her mobility.
I visit Helle towards the end of August. She seems more alert and positive about her illness. She tells me that her sister in Denmark has sent a gluten free diet, which Helle has been trying over the last couple of weeks. Helle says that she is feeling much better although there are occasions when she is still being sick.

I start my counselling course at the Pellin Centre in September. It is all women on the course and the course leader is also female. I am very comfortable with this group of women. The course is a Gestalt counselling course, which is mainly experiential, consisting of group work, working in pairs and practising our counselling skills in groups of four. We, therefore, quickly get to know each other very well. There are eighteen women on the course and all the women there are between their mid thirties and fifty years of age. I am now nearly forty. I discover that one third of this group of women have been sexually abused as children. Three of us experienced long term sexual abuse and the abusers were close members of the family (father, stepfather and brother). The other four women were sexually abused or assaulted in a one off incident by a mother's boyfriend, a teacher, a neighbour and one woman experienced an assault by a stranger in the park.

The next occasion when I go to visit Helle she tells me, "The consultant at Epsom hospital has visited me at home. He has recommended that I go into hospital for further checks as I am still losing weight and feeling weak."

Helle goes into hospital. Helle's son phones me and says that Helle had asked him to contact me and has asked for me to visit her in Epsom hospital as soon as possible. I go to visit Helle on Monday. I haven't seen her for two weeks. I go to the ward where her son told me she would be. He said that she was in a side ward but, as I approach her room, a nurse stops me and tells me that she has gone to theatre to have some tests carried out.

Helle's side ward is situated by a back door to the ward. I sit on the step and wait. Helle's son arrives and we wait together for Helle to be returned to the ward. We seem to sit there for ages. Helle's son talks about Helle, how it was for him growing up with her as his mum, he also talks about her work and how different her work is from his father's, his sister's and his own. We have waited about an hour and a half before Helle is pushed back onto the ward and into her room. She looks terrible, she is so thin and she has bruises scattered over her chest. Helle tells me it is where the doctors have tried to get a camera down into her stomach to see what was going on and what was causing her to lose so much weight. Helle's hair is hanging loosely around her shoulders. She normally wears her hair in a bun, so she looks different to me. Her son takes the flowers that I have brought and goes to put them in water. When he returns he switches on a radio that is in Helle's room. The voice on the radio is talking about road works on one of the 'A' roads. Helle says, "I hope that is finished before I get out of here, that's the road that I take to get me to L.C.P." I think how odd! You look so ill and I think that you might be dying and yet you're worrying about getting to work when you leave hospital.

I know that Helle is being given morphine for the pain that she is in and I think that this might be the reason for her thinking that she can return to work, or was she really going to get better? Helle goes on to tell her son and myself about her friend and colleague Joy visiting her and how she sent her out to buy her a bottle of red wine. Helle says, "They don't like me drinking in here but it makes my stomach feel better and I won't be told what to do." Typical Helle, I think to myself. I have to smile. She will not conform.

Helle's son leaves saying that he will be back later. When he has gone Helle beckons me to come and sit closer to her bed. She holds my hand and says, "Pam, it's time to say goodbye, it's time because I am not going to come out of this. Do you understand what I am telling you?"
I nod my head indicating that I know exactly what she is telling me. I lay my head on her chest. My head is spinning and the room is swimming around me. Helle strokes my hair and says, "I am so sorry, Pam. I am so sorry but I think it is better for you to experience this with me rather than on your own."
I brush Helle's hair for her and plump her pillow so that she is more comfortable. We spend some time chatting together before Helle's husband and daughter arrive for the evening visit. I have been there since 2pm. I say "Hello" to Helle's husband and her daughter, although I have never met her daughter before. Helle says, "No, don't go yet, all sit there together." She points to a place where she can see all three of us together. I sit there for about five minutes but I feel so uncomfortable that I say, "I really must go." I lean over Helle's bed to give her a kiss goodbye. She said quietly in my ear, "I knew that you would find it difficult to stay."

I tell Helle that I will be back to visit on the Wednesday of that week. I can't get to see her on Tuesday, as I have to make arrangements with work to take time off.

As I leave the hospital and walk to the train station, I feel numb. It all feels so unreal, this couldn't possibly be happening. I also feel so angry because, not being a member of the family, I can't ask for the information that I need to know. Why have they taken her off the gluten free diet? Why can't they get the camera into Helle's stomach?

The following day I meet with Mark, my Line Manager, and make arrangements to take leave on the Wednesday afternoon and all day on the Friday. I spend the rest of Tuesday functioning on automatic pilot. I am getting used to functioning this way, there are parts of myself that are split off, I can't handle what is happening, I am not able to cry and I spend long periods of time staring into space but seeing nothing, feeling nothing and thinking about nothing.
I go to bed on the Tuesday evening with all the lights on. I have slept with all the lights on since Beth left home. I am in my flat on my own. I wake up in the early hours of Wednesday morning. It feels like a cold gust of wind has flown through the window and penetrated through my bedclothes. I feel a cold shiver down my back and down my legs. I get up and go to the kitchen to get myself a glass of water. I look at the clock beside my bed. It reads 3.30 am. I don't think any more of it. I feel fine and go straight back to sleep.

I wake up, take a shower and start to iron some clothes to wear. The phone rings. It's Helle's daughter. She says, "I am so sorry to tell you that Helle died in the early hours of the morning."
I ask her what time this morning. She says, "She died at 3.30 this morning."

It seems to me that Helle had come to say goodbye when I woke up at 3.30 am.
I ask her daughter if I can attend Helle's funeral. She explains that the family want to keep it just for family members but that she will ask her father and get back to me.

I phone Beth and tell her that Helle has died. Beth comes around straight away. She helps me with my ironing and I go off to work. There are meetings that I need to cancel and other administrative tasks that can't be left. When I get to work someone who I don't know phones me. I speak to this woman. My voice sounds as if it is miles away. She asks, "Are you alright?" I tell her that someone close to me has died this morning. I know that I can't stay at work.

I go back home, I walk rather than catching the bus. The ground under my feet keeps moving. I am so pleased to get back home. I can only sit here. I don't know what to do with myself.
Helle's daughter phones me back a couple of days later. She tells me that I can go to the funeral, but they don't know when the funeral is going to be, as there has to be a post-mortem to establish the exact cause of Helle's death. She tells me that Val, Helle's friend and colleague, is also going to attend Helle's funeral and Val will let me know when and where the funeral will take place.

Valerie phones me a few days later and tells me that Helle's family has been told the post-mortem results. Valerie says, "Helle died from a complaint called celiac disease. This disease meant that Helle's system could not tolerate any wheat products. Helle also suffered from burst ulcers."

I think to myself: "Well, that's alright then, now the hospital can help Helle. Now that they know what is wrong with her they can make her better."

I am soon to be disillusioned of this thought as Valerie goes on to tell me the time, place and date of Helle's funeral.

Helle died on the 10th October 1990 and her funeral is taking place two weeks later. It is a horrible, damp, wet morning. It is such a bleak scene as I see the hearse carrying Helle's coffin driving up the driveway to the front of the church. There are no flowers. She wanted money to be donated to a charity. When we are inside the church Helle's family sit in the front. I sit a few rows back in between Valerie and Paul, who is also a colleague of Helle's from L.C.P. I am shivering and I comment to Paul about how cold it is. He says, "I think it has more to do with how you are feeling, Pam. It isn't really that cold." I feel rather protected, sitting between Valerie and Paul. I don't feel so alone.

After a very short service I go with Valerie to her house along with Joy and other members of WILL London. People are talking about Helle and their relationship with her. I find myself saying nothing. All that I think and feel stays inside me. Valerie and Joy suggest that a memorial service should be held for Helle, for all the people that Helle had known over the years who would have liked to have attended her funeral. Joy and Val are going to organise it and Val asks me to co-lead it with her. Helle's memorial will be carried out in the same way as we would run a WILL London workshop.

As I leave Valerie's house and am making my way home, the ground beneath my feet starts to move. I look at the traffic that is still moving and think to myself: "How can life still be going on?" I feel confused. It is as if I am having a nightmare that I haven't woken up from. I don't know how but I make my way home. A friend that I have made at one of the lesbian groups that I have been attending calls at my door and persuades me to go back to her house and sleep in her spare bedroom. I stay with Eva for a few days before returning home.

The first night at home since Helle's funeral, I drink a few glasses of wine. I think this will be better than sitting up half the night. I get to sleep about midnight and wake up again about 2am. I feel as if I am going mad, the room is swaying and I start to cry. My crying turns into deep sobs from deep inside of myself. This goes on for a good hour before I drift back to sleep.
The following morning, as I am going out to the shops, a neighbour stops me and asks me, "Did you hear that noise last night?" I look blankly at her. I don't know what she is talking about. She says, "That noise, it sounded like a baby sobbing, but we don't have any babies living in this block, do we?" I acknowledge that we don't and hurry past her. I remember me crying and feel so embarrassed. My family's words came back to me, "Don't cry and never cry. It's a sign of weakness to cry."

On the evening of Helle's memorial, I am pleased by how many people have attended. I have friends of mine there. Pat is there as is Claire B who I work with. Anna, the course leader from the Pellin institute, is also coming. I was a bit surprised when Anna told me that she had worked with Helle a few years ago and knew her well. It seems that Helle was well known and respected by a lot of people.

The memorial starts well and in true WILL London style people are asked to say whatever they want to say. Individuals talk about how they knew Helle and what they admired and liked about her. Then a young man stands up and says that he was a student of Helle's. He went on to say what a good experience he had having Helle as a teacher and he started to tell this group of people about a case that Helle had used with them. He described this person's history and how Helle had worked with this client. He was talking about me! I remember giving Helle permission to use our work with her students but this completely threw me. I just freeze. I am taken back in time. I am there back in Helle's consulting room. Joy steps in and takes over co-leading with Valerie.

CHAPTER NINE
NEW RELATIONSHIPS

A few days after the memorial, I drink a lot of wine and I am playing music, loudly. Felicity phones and asks, "Are you alright?" She then says, "No, you are not, are you?" She comes straight over, by which time I am sobbing from a place deep within me. Felicity comforts me for a while. She explains that she can't stay for long because she has to get back for her children. She doesn't want to leave me alone, so she phones Claire B who comes over with her partner John. They stay with me for a couple of days.

It is late October. Eva knocks on my door and suggests that we go for a walk in Waterlow Park. As we walk through the park gate, the vibrant colours of the autumn trees, lovely burnt oranges and deep reds, immediately strike me. Maybe I am seeing this beautiful world through Helle's eyes, as I have never noticed the autumn colours before. It is as if I am seeing it for the first time.
November comes and goes. I have my forty-first birthday. My birthdays have always been either a non-event or a painful reminder of how insignificant I have always felt. This leads to depressed thoughts of my father not wanting me and my mother wanting me dead before I had even been born. This birthday is a non-event, but at least I don't have to pretend to be happy. When my children were small, I felt that I had to make an effort. I forced myself to go with them to firework displays although I hated them with a passion.
When I was in the children's home I have no memory of my birthday. Perhaps because it was fireworks night, my birthday was overshadowed and when I returned home I was given fireworks as birthday presents but they were for the whole family to enjoy. I had nothing for myself.

I carry on with my counselling course and I feel supported by the other women on the course. My first grandchild is due to be born sometime in the early part of December. I am at the hospital with Beth when she is told that the baby has moved position: she has turned and is lying sideways in Beth's tummy instead of the normal birth position. The hospital tells Beth that she will need to have a Caesarean section rather than giving birth normally. Beth says, "I'm scared, mum."

"I am sure everything will be O.K., Beth. I will be there with you and it will be alright." But I do feel frightened for both Beth and her baby.

Andrew, Beth's partner, says, "I can't stay, I can't stand the sight of blood."

"I will be there with you, don't worry," I say.

Monday morning, the 10th of December 1990, Beth goes into hospital. Beth is given an epidural injection into her spine; she wants to be awake for the birth of her child. I am asked to put on a surgical gown. They take her into the delivery room and I follow. I stand beside my daughter's bed as the doctor makes an incision into Beth's stomach. Suddenly, Beth screams out in pain, "It hasn't worked. I can feel everything."

The epidural hasn't worked. I feel a wave of fear as I am swiftly guided out of the room and Beth is given an anaesthetic. Everything happens with great speed, there is no time to ask what is happening or protest about being guided out of the room. Within ten seconds other hospital staff have entered the delivery room and I watch helplessly through the window of the adjacent room as my granddaughter is born.

The baby is gently given to the paediatrician, who holds the baby closely to her, almost protecting her from the shock of being born. The paediatrician then examines the tiny baby before she places her in a cot and wheels her out

to me. I am holding Beth's new baby in my arms as Beth wakes up from the anaesthetic. I say, "You have a lovely baby girl, Beth".
Beth, who is still very drowsy, says: "I know I'm a girl mum, I know."
As she regains her senses, we laugh about her reaction.

After a few days, Beth leaves the hospital with her baby. She comes to see me at home and tells me that she has registered her baby's birth and that she has decided to call her Lucy Helle.
Lucy is a beautiful, dark haired, olive skinned baby with huge brown eyes. I am swept away by her perfection and the feelings of love that engulf me. It reminds me of the feelings I had for my own babies when they were born. I am very touched and honoured that Beth has called the baby Lucy Helle. I am mindful of the powerful impact that Helle has had on my life and Beth did this for me.
This event helps me to think about how I took time to build up a meaningful relationship with Helle and how painful it has been to say goodbye and how much I miss her. And yet here is a new life, a baby granddaughter. It is going to be a wonderful experience for me getting to know this little person called Lucy Helle. I baby-sit for Beth whenever the opportunity is offered and, by the time she is six months old, Lucy is coming to stay with me overnight.

I am still uncertain about my sexuality. I have tried two, very short-lived relationships. One of the lesbian students on the course says in the large group, "There are four and a half lesbians on this course."
One of the other women asks, "What do you mean four and a half lesbians? Where do you get the half from?"
The student who has made the comment looks at me and says, "Pam's the half, because she can't decide." I can see the funny side of this comment.

A year has passed since Helle's death and my dreaded birthday is approaching. I go out to the London Lesbian and Gay Club in Farringdon with a group of women. I catch a glimpse of a woman who is sitting on the edge of a table talking to someone that I know. I look and notice her gorgeous colouring as I see her sideways on. She has short chestnut coloured hair, a handsome woman with boyish looks. I make my way over to be introduced. Her name is Clare and, as she talks to me, I note that her complexion is English rose, she has green eyes and she is tall with long legs. We talk for a while and she tells me it is her birthday on the 4th of November. It is mine on the fifth. I invite her to my house along with a group of other women to a party that I have been persuaded to give.

Clare comes along and we spend most of the evening talking with one another. We seem to have a lot in common. Clare is a probation officer. She is on a psychotherapy course. This gives us a lot to share. We meet again at the birthday party of a friend. Once more we spend most of the evening together. I have to leave early because I am feeling very ill.

I am ill with a virus that seems to go on forever. It is very annoying because I invite Clare over to my home for a meal; the plan is to go out after our meal but I can't go out because I can't shake off the virus that eventually turns into a chest infection.

I question my illness, "Was this virus exacerbated by it being so close to the anniversary of Helle's death?" It is always difficult to know when I am ill whether it is physical or psychosomatic.

By Christmas I am well again. Clare and I go out to a gay club. For the first time, we kiss and she spends the night with me on Christmas Eve. I spend Christmas day with my son, daughter and granddaughter and I go to Clare's home on the Boxing Day. Over the next few weeks we are together most of the time. I enjoy her company and I love to be with her. I am in love. I have never experienced this before. I never had these feelings with Simon. In the evenings when I have finished work, I can't wait to see her. Clare and I decide to live together and she moves in with me, renting her own home to a friend.

I haven't talked to Jay or Beth about my sexuality. It didn't seem relevant to do so until I was sure. When Clare moves in I am sure and both my children need to know because I hope Clare is going to be my partner and is going to play a big part in my life. I am hoping that she will also be part of my children's life. When I tell Beth, she is delighted. She says, "Well, I think that is so cool, it's great". Jay is a little more guarded. He says "I don't understand it but if this relationship makes you happy, mum, and Clare is company for you, then that's great. I'm perfectly O.K. with you being with her."

Clare gets to know both Beth and Jay. She gets on very well with both of them and has a very close relationship with Lucy, who now stays with us every other weekend.

As I feared, Beth's relationship with Andrew ends and Beth now lives and has to manage as a single parent.

I am so happy, feeling high. I find I can talk to Clare about anything and she is equally open with me. We are soul mates. The one thing I was afraid of talking about was the sexual acting out when I was an adolescent. I eventually gather the courage to tell her and to my amazement Clare calmly says, "But that sort of behaviour is common with girls who have been sexually abused and is part and parcel of the abuse. Don't let it play on your mind."

I feel greatly relieved. I had feared that Clare, as a Probation officer, might have been judgemental and she might have seen me as soiled goods.

Clare was sad and concerned about all the distress it caused me and made it clear that I could talk to her about anything.
We have a lovely holiday together in Portugal where we talk and laugh together. We decide that we want to spend the rest of our lives together. We plan a commitment ceremony and invite Jay, Beth and Lucy, a lot of my friends and colleagues and Clare's friends from her course, her boss and other friends of hers. It is a wonderful, memorable day, when Clare and I make promises to one another witnessed by those who are dear to us.

I finish my counselling course and, although I have got a lot from it and it supported me in working through Helle's death, Helle was right about the Pellin course not being a recognised one and it hasn't enabled me to change my career from social worker to counsellor. The Pellin course isn't sufficient in as much as I cannot become accredited by any of the recognised accrediting bodies such as The British Association for Counsellors and Psychotherapists (B.A.C.P.) or United Kingdom Counsel for Psychotherapists (U.K.C.P.). I am working with some clients from home and I am receiving supervision from Anna, the Pellin tutor. I also work in a voluntary capacity as a counsellor with MIND. This contract is for two years. I receive monthly group supervision. I feel that I am competent to do short term work with clients, but I lack the theory and the skills to work on more complex and deeper problems.

CHAPTER TEN
THERAPY WITH SUE AT L.A.P.P.

I am still working for Islington Social Services. Both Clare and I live in Islington and have now been together for some time. I give it a lot of thought and talk through with Clare the possibility of going onto another training course. Clare suggests that I apply to The London Association of Primal Psychotherapists (LAPP). Clare has herself just completed a psychotherapy course with this organisation and is working through completing enough client hours to become accredited with U.K.C.P.

In order to be permitted to get on to this course, I am required to undergo a training psychotherapy. I think that I have worked through most of my childhood issues although there are times when I become depressed or irrationally angry with Clare. The anger occurs if Clare is ever late home for whatever reason. I rage at her, "Where have you been? I thought that something had happened to you. Why didn't you let me know?"
Clare replies, "Pam, I was kept at work. I couldn't let you know. What is this about?"
But there is no reassuring me, I feel so anxious and distraught. I can't bear the thought of losing her.
Clare is quite pleased that I am going to return to therapy because she thinks that clearly there are still unresolved issues from my childhood.

I apply to L.A.P.P. I am soon offered an appointment with a psychotherapist called Sue. My meeting goes well. Sue asks me about my personal history and when it comes to the end of the meeting, she says that she thinks that she has time in her schedule to see me as a client.

I receive a letter confirming my place on the course. L.A.P.P. is set up so that there are three rooms with cloth covered, mattress sized, oblongs of foam covering the whole of the floor area and similar oblongs standing along the walls to about three feet high. There are a number of cushions and clients are encouraged to use the room and the cushions in order to help them express their feelings and to make themselves feel comfortable enough to enable them to work in safety

Sue sends me a letter with my first appointment date. I arrive early. I wait outside the building where I cannot be seen until my watch shows that it is my appointment time. This reminds me that I waited where I could not be seen when I went to school as a child and at various times when I had appointments with senior management staff at Islington.

Sue is about the same age as me. She is petite with dark hair and dark eyes and well spoken. For the first few months or so when working with her, I talk about my childhood, my children and my work. Sue points out that I speak in a rational manner and I am like a social worker reading a report on someone else. She doesn't feel that I am talking about myself in a feeling way. Instead, I am very distant. When I leave the session I think to myself, "I'm not going to show myself up. I can't and won't feel those awful love feelings that I felt for Helle."

In the next session with Sue she suggests that I do some drawings with her. I protest saying, "I am useless at drawing."
Sue says, "It doesn't matter whether you can draw or not, Pam. You can draw matchstick men if you want to. All I want you to do is to draw whatever comes into your head.

Don't think about it too much; just draw whatever comes into your mind."

I agree to do the drawing. My first drawing is of a brick wall with Sue on one side and me on the other. Sue asks me why there might be such a distance between us. I tell her that I am scared, scared that I might have feelings that get me into trouble. I tell her about my love feelings for Helle and how I also had these same feelings in my teenage years towards my mother. I say, "Other teenage girls had crushes on boys. I wasn't interested in boys. The only person that I had passionate love feelings for was my mother. Before my mother I loved Mummy Robins, from the children's home. These feelings have always got me into trouble and I have to control them."

Sue calmly says that this is something that obviously needs to be worked on.

In the next session we use drawings, too. I draw two or three aeroplanes exploding in the sky. This reminds me of the aeroplanes that I drew for the psychiatrist at St Bartholomew's Hospital when I was a teenager. I tell Sue about this and say, "I think this is about when I was abandoned in the children's home."

I look at the drawings again and say, "Oh no! They are not exploding aeroplanes. They are exploding penises."

Sue says, "Yes, they do look like that."

Sue asks me to talk about where that image came from. I think perhaps from Uncle Harry's sexual abuse of me. Many images and memories come to my mind in quick succession and I manage to push them away.

In another session with Sue, I draw a picture of a garden with trees and leaves and flowers. I also draw a woman's face in the sky. I say, "This was how I saw my mother when I was little: a mummy in the sky. Had I been told by staff that my mummy was dead and lived in the sky? I don't know. All I know is that this is the image that I can always remember."

Sue asks me if I have any photographs of me as a child. "I have a few, not many, maybe five or six." I take the photos that I have with me to the next session. I lay them out one by one on the floor and tell Sue what I know about them or remember of them. One photo is of a little girl of about three or four holding hands with two older boys. They are all dressed in swimsuits and they are standing on a pebble beach. I feel a pang of sadness. I say to Sue in a far away voice, "That's me and my two brothers. We must have been on holiday with the children's home but I don't even remember going on holiday while I was in care."

The next photo is a small torn photo of a little girl in a pushchair; bigger children surround her. I tell Sue in that far away voice, "They said that I was backward. I couldn't walk. I think that I had just moved from the nursery to the children's home."

There are two school photos of me, one of when I was about seven. The picture shows a girl sitting with a book in front of her. I say to Sue, "I don't know why I have a book in front of me, I couldn't read. I still couldn't read that well when I went to secondary school."

The other school photo is of a girl in a school uniform; she is about eleven years old and she has a slight smile on her lips. I say, "She looks alright. How can she look alright when she wasn't alright?"

Sue says, "Look at the eyes of yourself in the photograph, they look worried and uncertain. You were very small for your age."

I lay down the next photograph. It is of a small girl holding hands with, and looking at, two boys. The three children in the photo are well groomed. They are standing in front of a chain link fence. The little girl has a ribbon in her curly blond hair, my brother Dennis looks worried and my brother Joe looks happy. I explain to Sue, "We must have gone home for the weekend from the children's home, except it isn't home. The picture must have been taken outside of Aunty Rachel's house."

Memories, bad memories, start to run through my head; Joe has stolen money and is being caned for it by Uncle Harry. Everything inside me slows down. With these memories everything inside me seems to stop still. Time stops still. I feel alone in the room.

I quickly lay down the last photograph on the floor. It is of a girl (me). I am about five years old and I am lying on top of my stepfather, who is on a sun bed. My mother has put me there. I remember lying rigidly on top of him. I feel a huge rage swelling up inside myself. I lunge at the photos. Sue leans over to protect them. She says, "No, No. What is it that you want to do, Pam?"

I say, "I hate 'her'. I hate 'her'. See, she gets me into trouble. I just want to destroy 'her'. Tear 'her' up, tear 'her up and get rid of 'her'."

Sue says, "No, I can't let you do that but if you must tear something up I will give you some paper to tear up".

She sweeps the photos into her hands and produces some paper, which I savagely tear into shreds. Sue puts the pieces of paper into an envelope and she tells me that it is all right, I haven't destroyed anything and she will keep the torn up pieces of paper safely in the office. We talk about Sue keeping the photographs safely in the office as well. This seems a good idea; the photos are kept at LAPP.

One day in August 1995 Clare receives a phone call from her brother in Sussex. He tells Clare that her father has died earlier that morning. We travel down to Sussex later that day and stay in Clare's auntie's caravan. The caravan is situated in a little village called Ferring. Ferring is by the coast and not far from Clare's parents' house. Clare sorts out and makes all the arrangements for her father's funeral as Clare's mother has Alzheimer's disease and is not able to make any of the arrangements. I find myself thinking about Clare's father and other male relatives in Clare's family. I am struck by how few of the men that I have met in my life are good. Mark, who was my line manager at Islington Social Services, has been very supportive and he is a gentle intelligent man. Clare's father, brothers and her uncle Richard also have these qualities. Whenever I meet them I always feel shocked and deeply moved by them as my experiences of men have been so brutal and unkind. Even during the years that I spent with Simon, I didn't experience him as being loving and gentle. He was distant and rather cold towards me. He wanted sex, not a close caring relationship. Perhaps he hadn't had enough good parenting himself. His own father didn't show any soft feelings and Simon's mother was not the touchy feely type. The men in Clare's family are certainly different from the men that I have grown up with. They are gentle and kind and they like and respect women and respect all the other people around them.

I support Clare through her father's funeral and we stay at on for a few days to be with Clare's mum.

I talk to Sue about my feelings towards men and my relationship with my brothers. I seem to come away from therapy feeling as if I have been hit over the head with a hammer. It is as if I keep returning to a different time, a different space, but it is as if it is happening today. I am either seeing 'Her' or watching what is happening as if I am watching a play on the stage. Or I am one of the actors taking part.

It is clear that there is a split, a part of myself that is not integrated with the adult part of me. I refer to the child me as 'her' or 'she'. I do not see her as me so that I have separated the adult me from what happened to Pam the child. This protects me from carrying the very painful feelings which are kept in therapy. When I say 'her' and 'she' I am referring to myself. This is a move forward from the time when I worked with Helle because I then called the child in me 'it' as if I was an object.

Overwhelming feelings take me over and after each session I have to get myself together, go to work and manage a team of staff who are working with a vulnerable client group. I start to see Sue twice weekly, once is not enough! Clare is always there for me. I feel that I can always talk to Clare. Once or twice I use drink to numb the pain, as I did in the past, but I now find that using drink doesn't work any more and I really need to go through the feelings and hope that I will come out the other side.

Clare and I go for a short break and stay at Clare's aunties' caravan. As we are walking along the riverbank, making our way down to the sea, I become very panicky. I am convinced that we are going to get lost. My anxiety becomes huge. Clare reminds me about other occasions when we have been walking in the countryside, either in England or abroad, when I became convinced that something dreadful was going to happen and I felt terrified. When I go for my session with Sue I tell her about what has happened. She encourages me to tell her more. I go back to the past, "I am at the camp in Romford. I can smell the paraffin oil that is used to light the oil lamps. I can see long grass. He has me by the hand, he is taking me somewhere."

The picture of me lying on top of Uncle Harry comes vividly into my mind.

"His trousers are undone, his trousers are always undone. He is pinching the tops of 'her' legs. 'She' can't stand it."

"He pushes 'her' off of him and he says, 'Dirty little bitch. You dirty little bitch'. He pushes 'her' towards 'her' mother and says, 'Clean her up, the dirty little bitch has wet herself'."

I tell Sue, "But my mother never washes 'her'. It's always him that washes 'her'. He gets a metal tub and stands 'her' in it whist he roughly washes 'her' hair and scrubs 'her' body clean."

I sit up from my lying position. Sue is sitting beside me. I ask her if I can hold her hand. Sue holds my hand and we talk about what has just happened. Sue gently points out that when I talk about "She can't stand it", it's me who couldn't stand it. Sue says, "Try saying 'I can't stand it'. She is part of you."

I tell Sue, "He often pinched the tops of my legs, he would start by tickling them and then he pinched them until it was unbearable. When I got back to the children's home, my mother told the staff that I bruised the tops of my legs when I fell onto the cross bar or when riding one of my brother's bikes. It was a lie."

LAPP is moving premises. The new premises have a waiting area. There is much the same set up in the rooms that I use and am accustomed to in the old building.

My next appointment with Sue is at the new premises in Swains Lane. Clare and I drive there in the car. As I approach the front entrance, I see one of the psychotherapists and another man standing by the entrance. I feel paralysed. A wave of panic sweeps over me. I return to the car and tell Clare that I can't go in there. I ask Clare if she can go and tell Sue that I can't make it today. Sue comes out of the building and says, "Come on, I will walk in with you."

She has already asked the men to go inside the building away from the entrance. As I walk into the new L.A.P.P. building, I feel like I am walking through a fog. I don't know how I make it into the room but I do and I collapse onto the mattress and cover my eyes. I cannot explain why I have reacted in this way although I do know that I have experienced this type of thing before.

It seems that in every therapy session that I go to, there are always flashbacks coming up, some of these flashbacks are memories that I have dealt with before, only this time there is a different slant on them, or I remember people or the place in more detail. Sue asks me, "What is happening, Pam?"
I say, "I don't know."
My mind is like a camera that flashes through frame after frame in quick succession. Then the camera settles on one memory.
I am back there, I can see 'her' walking down the balcony; 'she' looks about twelve years old. 'She' takes the key, which is hanging on a piece of string inside the letterbox. 'She' turns the key in the lock and opens the front door. Everything is happening in slow motion. 'She' stops. My mind freezes.
Sue asks me, "What can you see? Describe everything in detail."
I say, "I love you, I love you, Sue".
Sue asks, "What's happening?"
I reply, "I need to feel safe. I love you. It will be alright because I love you."
"He is here. His breakfast things are on the table. 'She' has frozen. 'She' can't move. He calls 'her'. He has run 'her' a bath. He washes 'her'. He is touching 'her'. Oh my God, it hurts, it hurts."
Sue says, "What is he doing to you?"
"He has folded 'her' up into a ball on the sofa. My head, my head hurts. He has Vaseline; he puts it inside 'her'."
A voice deep inside me says, "Shut up, you little bitch. Shut your fucking mouth or I will shut it for you." I am

punching myself, shouting, "Shut up, you fucking little bitch."

Sue says "Pam, no, come on, you are not to hurt yourself." She puts a large cushion between my fists and my face.

I continue to punch and shout for a long time. The scene changes: "'She' is back at school staring out of the window. It's crying inside, 'she' wants to die. 'She' feels dirty and 'she' wants to die."

The scene changes again. "'She' has met her mother at the bus stop; 'she' carries her mother's bag. Her mother is happy with 'her' because 'she' pleased Uncle Harry."

Sue asks me to mentally come back into the room. She says, "Look around you. Look at the room."

I ask if I can hold her hand. Sue holds my hand and I say, "I love you, it will be alright because I love you."

Sue and I talk about what happens in the sessions. We piece it together. Sue tells me that when I am talking about 'her' or 'she' I am talking about myself. She says try and say 'I' or 'ME'.

I tell Clare about the session as we go home and I say, "I wonder what my fear of entering L.A.P.P. was about."

Clare points out, "Present day happenings can trigger off old memories and the feelings belonging to those memories become attached to the present day events. It is possible that the experience of entering L.A.P.P. triggered off the memory of going into the flat where Uncle Harry abused you. So, it was that fear that you were feeling when you tried to go into L.A.P.P. and that was the memory that was close enough to the surface for it to come up in your session."

What Clare was saying felt right but my mind was still very muddled after my session and it took a little while before I could digest and make sense of what had happened.

From the time when the flashbacks started I am unable to look at Sue, I hide my face and my eyes behind my hands and this continues in every session.

The words "I love you, I love you" make me feel better and help me to push away painful feelings. They are part of a defence mechanism, which has helped me to survive as a small child using a fantasy of an ideal mother in the sky that cared for me. I tended to unconsciously perceive kind carers, teachers, social workers and when I started therapy, therapists, as this ideal mother.

In the next session I tell Sue how vivid it all was in the last session. I sit on the padded floor with my hand hiding my eyes and tell Sue what I can remember from the last session.

"The sofa, I can remember the sofa in detail: dark brown leatherette, a dark brown sofa with big chunky arms. That is the sofa that turned into my bed at nighttime. How could the three of them be coming into my bedroom at night time, without them ever bumping into each other or them not knowing what the other two were doing? It just doesn't make sense."

Sue asks me what happened when they climaxed. "Did they clean the mess up? Did I get up and clean the mess up?"

I say, "No, they climaxed onto my tummy and left me there. No, I never got out of bed, I was too frightened to move."

Sue said, "The mess must have been on the sheets."

I pause in thought; then I say, "Yes, it must have been. The same with my knickers when he sent me back to school."

Sue says, "Pam, your mother must have known what was happening."

My head is spinning. I hadn't thought about my mother knowing. I always told myself that she didn't know. This unthinkable thought stayed with me for weeks and for many weeks distressed me.

Sue tells me that the training course has been postponed for a period of time because LAPP hasn't managed to get enough students to enrol for the course to make the course viable. Tears roll down my cheeks. I can't believe it. It seems like the end of my world. I feel betrayed and let down. Sue has let me down and she can't make everything all right. I know in reality that these things happen, it's life, but for this session something inside me feels broken. Sue can't put it right.

In my life outside of therapy, work is heavy going. More pressure is being placed on managers to be responsible for budgets. Staffing levels are being cut and training courses for managers are mainly around personnel procedures. Strategies for dealing with staff lateness and sickness are a priority as are staff's appraisal and development procedures.

Senior staff that I have respected for many years have already left or are leaving the service. There are not many people left working in Islington who I feel that I can trust or talk to. Clare and I support each other, as Clare is experiencing much the same in the probation service at this time.

Clare is feeling very tired which is unlike her. When she hears that the Probation Service is offering early retirement on advantageous conditions she does not think that this will apply to her or that she will have enough pension to be able to afford to retire and doesn't apply at this time. Shortly after this she is diagnosed as having Hashimoto's Thyroiditis, a disease of the immune system in which the immune system attacks the thyroid gland. She is told that she will need to take thyroid replacement therapy for the rest of her life. Once she starts taking her thyroid replacement tablets, she becomes alert, energized and motivated to look into the matter of early retirement and what is on offer. Clare makes enquires and finds that the terms being offered are quite beneficial and she will be able to afford to retire. She takes early retirement and this enables her to build up her psychotherapy practice.

CHAPTER ELEVEN
TRAINING AND THERAPY WITH SUE

Over many sessions of therapy with Sue, I find myself telling her about the ordeal of what happened to me if I refused to have sex with Uncle Harry. I say, "I never directly said 'No' to him, I just didn't go home from school at lunch times, I wandered the streets; I misbehaved and made sure that I got kept behind at school at the end of the day."

I sigh, "When I eventually got home, Uncle Harry ignored me and when my mother got home I hadn't made my brothers' beds, their room wasn't tidy, the breakfast dishes hadn't been home from work. He told her that I hadn't completed all the chores that I was expected to do around the washed up, the shopping wasn't done and I hade not prepared the vegetables for tea."

I say to Sue, "I'm like fucking Cinderella, aren't I?"

A voice from inside me says, "Useless bitch, fucking useless bitch. I hate her."

I attempt to punch my face. Sue puts a cushion between my face and my punching fists. I punch the cushion that is up against my face and then turn and crouch on my knees and punch another cushion that was at the back of me shouting, "I hate you. I fucking hate you."

When I have run out of steam Sue brings me mentally back into the room. We talk about what has happened. I tell Sue that the rage was towards the useless child and then my rage turned towards my mother.

I continue to tell Sue how I resented all the chores that I was expected to do. "There were numerous other jobs that were deemed to be my responsibility, depending on what day of the week it was, for example, Wednesday was bagwash day and I should have hung up the clean clothes that came back from the laundry in the drying room, that was situated along the balcony from our flat. If it was a

Thursday then I was expected to get home from school and start the ironing."

If the work wasn't done, my mother looked at me with disgust; she would wail in a whining voice, "I can't cope with this. I am at work all day. Why do you do this to me? You make me ill. You are always causing me trouble."

Another image comes to mind; I recall how I stood by my mother in the kitchen, which was tiny, whilst she dished out the evening meal that uncle Harry had cooked. It is as if am back there, "The evening meal is fatty lamb, which uncle Harry has brought home from Smithfield meat market. With the lamb, which is swimming in fat, are over cooked stewed greens and plain boiled potatoes."

As I am telling and reliving this, an image comes into my mind. I say, "It's like a scene from a Dickens novel, I can see myself carrying the plates of food into the sitting room and giving them out as my mother has directed me. I feel so resentful as I notice that my brothers get more food than me. I mumble, "It's not fair, it's just not fair." I don't dare to speak out directly. Uncle Harry says, "What are you mumbling about?"

I mumble, "Nothing", putting my head down.

My mother comes in from the kitchen and says, "Nothing, nothing. You fucking little bitch."

She smacks me across the face so hard that the force of her smack sends me flying across the room. I feel a dizziness in my head and a ringing in my ears as I am telling Sue in the voice of a child.

I continue telling Sue, "I eat my meal in silence. My brothers and myself are told to eat the fat on the lamb, even if it does make us heave. After the meal, I wash up and then wait in the bedroom to be punished. Uncle Jack, the stick, is brought into the bedroom from the sitting room. I am stripped from the waist down and am beaten."

My mind fast-forwards like a videotape and it skips the part where I am beaten. I can't tell Sue any details about the beating. "I don't feel any pain. I just see huge welts on my skin where he has hit me. I am standing in the bedroom where I have been left to get myself dressed and to think about what I have done wrong. I think about nothing. I go into another world and time passes without me noticing."

Whilst still emotionally in the past, I tell Sue how the time frame changes in my head, "I am now sitting in the corner. 'They', my brothers, are not allowed to talk to me. I can see 'her' sitting there, in the corner. I can also see another image of 'her' hovering above 'her own' head. There is a part of 'her' that has left 'her' sitting in the corner. I can see Uncle Harry handing sweets around, bars of chocolate. One for my mother, one for Dennis and Uncle Harry eats the remaining four bars."
He says, "None for you."
As Dennis walks by to go to the toilet he kicks me in the back and says, "Slag, fucking slag."
Sue asks, "What can we do to help that little girl who is you?"
My head is spinning and I say, "I don't know."
Sue says, "I think that the adult part of you and I should go and get her out of that place. Let's bring her out to a place of safety."
In imagination I watch as Sue and the adult part of myself walk into the sitting room. The room that belongs to the past, so many years ago, now looks as real as ever in my mind as it did then. Sue takes this child by the hand and leads her out of the room. The adult part of me follows.
Before the end of the session Sue and I talk about what has happened and she asks me what I have made of my reliving of this event.
I wonder out loud, "Why was my mother more caring towards my brothers? Was I bad? Was it my fault?"

"How can we make sense of madness, Pam? Uncle Harry reminds me of a commandant in a Nazi concentration camp. For him it was all about power and brutality to all three children. From what I can see your brothers came out of this more damaged than you. You could say that they sold their souls, in that they went along with him in order to survive. As for your mother, none of you actually got anything worthwhile, even your brothers got the crumbs from the table."

The image of me sitting in the corner comes up more than once in therapy sessions. Once again I am back in the flat, in memory, watching the scene as it unfolds in my inner eye. I say, "This punishment of sitting in the corner goes on for such a long time, sometimes weeks. Then when Uncle Harry decides that it is time to end this part of the punishment, he sends the rest of the family out of the sitting room for the evening, he sits me up at the dining room table and sits by my side. It always happens at seven in the evening. If 7pm comes and goes, then I know that I have another evening of sitting in the corner. The rest of the family have left the room without asking any questions. My brothers go out of the flat and my mother busies herself in the small kitchen. They never come back into the room again until uncle Harry says so.
Uncle Harry talks at me. He tells me that I am bad. He says, "Go on, tell me that you are bad. I want to hear it."
"I have to admit it. I tell him that I am bad."
"He says that I am bad like my father and Joe. He always says that Joe is like his father."
I pause and say, "I think that Joe probably looks like our father and I certainly look like Joe."

When I am first piecing this part of the punishment together with Sue I tell her, "I can't remember the words he used to say to me. I can see him talking at me, but I can't hear what he is saying, I can see a part of me leaving my body. He talks at me for what seems like hours."

I begin to feel numb and dead inside, then I feel icy cold almost an icy cold rage. "Sue, Sue," I say urgently, "Knives come into my mind; I can see Uncle Harry with his meat knives."

Then I hear his words, "You tell and I'll slit your throat. You tell, you little bitch, and I will cut your tongue out."

"He keeps going on and on at 'her'."

He asks, "Who do you talk to? What do you say?"

"He tells 'her' endlessly that he knows all about 'her', he can see 'her' at all times. 'She' feels frozen with fear and 'she' believes every word."

Every time I refer to my self in the past I always call me 'Her' or 'She.' Once again, Sue challenges me about this.

When Sue asks me to bring my mind back into the room I suddenly realise that this ritualistic punishment of caning at a set time, being sent to Coventry by all the family, the tormenting by my brothers, the rest of the family being given sweets to eat whilst I am left out, and Uncle Harry talking at me and threatening me, was a pattern that was continuously put into practice over a period of three or four years, every time I didn't have sex with him.

It is only now that I can see it as a ritual. It takes me weeks to understand why I have forgotten or haven't seen it before, this pattern, that is now so clear.

Clare and I decide that we want to move from our flat in Islington and move south of the river. The houses that are in our price range are in the borough of Merton. Clare wants to build up a private practice from home. She also continues with the clients that she sees at LAPP. I plan to travel to work and therapy by using the Northern Line tube network. Moving isn't an easy decision as I am going away from both Beth and my granddaughter Lucy. I am also moving away from Jay and his partner and the area where I have lived almost all my life.

Just before the move I start to become anxious about moving to an area that I don't know. The shops aren't nearby. How often do the buses run? How will I cope with the tube journey to work, to therapy and to visit my children and grandchild? The first few weeks, after moving to our new house, are awful. I tell Clare that I hate it and moving was the worst mistake that I have ever made. I blame Clare and at times I become very angry with her. I dread the tube journeys. I think that something terrible is going to happen. It feels as if I have been taken to a place that I don't know. I don't know anyone in the area and I fear that I will be left alone and unsupported.

Through therapy and talking to Clare, I realise that these feelings mostly belong in my childhood. They are about all the moves that happened: being taken into care as a baby, moving from the nursery to the children's home, the move from the children's home to my mother's flat at Manor House and the move from Wellingborough to London, which triggered off my last breakdown. Clare points out that the words I use, "I have made a terrible mistake," are the same words that I used when I left Wellingborough.

Shortly after moving home, the psychotherapy course at L.A.P.P finally starts. I acknowledge to myself that the course being delayed was probably the best thing that could have happened for me, as I wasn't ready. I needed more time in therapy without the course intruding into much needed work that had to be done.

I feel nervous and excited. The course is held at L.A.P.P. on Monday and Tuesday evenings. On the evening of the first day of the course, all four students meet with the course co-ordinator. Her name is Marsha. She explains the structure of the first year of the course. There are lectures to attend, baby observations and a training group therapy.

The baby observations consist of a year of observing a mother and baby in their home. We are required to write process recordings of the baby's development and the interaction and dynamics between mother and child, also the interaction between family members. As students we have to find a family who are willing to allow psychotherapy students to observe them. I find a family quite quickly. My long-standing friend Claire B, who has started a family with her partner John, has experienced being observed by a student from another psychotherapy course. She found the experience rewarding and has contact with a new mum who is willing to be observed.

Kay is a young woman from Devon. She is married with a four and a half year old son and she has just given birth to a baby girl. They live in Haringey. The family lives in a two-bedroom housing association flat, situated on the fifth floor. There is no lift and it almost kills me when I climb the stairs to their flat every Monday at 4pm.

Every other week students take it in turns to read out their recordings of the process of the observation to the rest of the group so that the seminar leader and the other students can make comments and add their observations.

Before the course starts, Sue tells me, "I think that it is important that you are able to tell me about any thoughts or feelings that come up for you during your training. Therapy is my main concern and the course, although it is important, comes second to me than working with you in therapy."

I find myself telling Sue, shortly after the course has started, about feelings that I am finding difficult to deal with. The feelings first come up in the training group. "I can't understand why I find it so difficult and painful to be with the other three students," I tell Sue.

"I have never found it so difficult in other training groups that I have been involved with, for example WILL London and The Pellin Institute. I have also been involved in training groups at work and with MIND."

Sue asks me, "What is different about this group of people?"

I tell her, "I don't know. I have always got on with most people in the other groups but in this group it sometimes feels like I am an outsider. I feel different, not as good as the rest of them. I feel like an alien, Sue. None of the other four students have had any of the same sorts of problems that I have experienced."

One of the students is Maltese. She is my age and Clare and I already know her. One is German and a little younger than I am and the third woman is Greek and she is very young, the same age as my daughter Beth. I feel that the dynamics between us are difficult, to say the least. We all come from different cultures. Two of the women are engaged in a constant battle. The male leader of the training therapy group seems unable to hold or explore the anger between these two group members. The third student, who is the youngest, seems very inexperienced in life and she remains very quiet for most of the time. I find the two members of the group irritating. They are constantly arguing and sniping at one another about the same thing, and the group leader does not intervene in any way, so nothing is resolved.

As I continue telling Sue about this, I begin to realise that I find that the constant going on by these two people triggers off memories of Uncle Harry keeping on at me. Although I am not the subject of the argument, I feel that I am back there in that flat sitting in the corner. There is a lot of rivalry for attention from the tutors and this reminds me of the children's home where getting the attention of the staff was difficult.

On one occasion one of the group members is upset and is talking about having spent two weeks in hospital as a baby. The group leader, at some point, makes a comment to me, that her experience of going to hospital for two weeks is similar to me being in care. I am furious and can't see any relationship between two weeks in hospital and six years in care.

I begin to feel envious about the better life that the other three students have had as children. I also resent that they are able to talk about their early life so freely, when I find it so difficult. Sometimes we meet in the café for coffee before the course starts. The other three students talk about their extended families. I feel clumsy, awkward and I withdraw into myself. I remain silent. The group might feel like a family and I am the only one who has been sexually abused. Here too I am Cinderella who cannot talk about my experiences, whilst the others can.

I take all of this to therapy and work on it with Sue. I rage about the unfairness of life. Sue takes me through these painful feelings and memories step by step. She gets me to punch into a cushion. This isn't easy for me, as I fear that I will go insane with these powerful overwhelming feelings. Sue is persistent and, after I have punched into a cushion for a few minutes, my rage takes over.

Sue says, "Use some words, Pam."

No words will come. I just kept punching into the cushion.

Sue says, "If you can't use words, try and make sounds."

I try and small oh, oh sounds come out as I continue to punch into the cushion. I can hear Sue saying, "Louder, louder, Pam."

My punching on the cushions becomes faster as the words come tumbling out. I say, "I hate you, I hate you, fucking bastard, I hate you. Get off of me. Get off my back. Oh, he's heavy on my back. Oh, it hurts. It hurts."

Sue places her hand gently on my back. Deep sobs from way deep inside myself come gushing out, my whole body hurts all over and the sobbing goes on and on. The words

that follow are "I'm sorry, mummy, I'm so sorry. Please don't hate me, please don't leave me."
As the sobbing subsides, Sue brings me back to the present and I can tell her what memories have gone flashing through my mind. Sue also tells me what she has seen and we piece it together like a jigsaw puzzle.
This is the first time that I have been able to express any anger against Uncle Harry. Perhaps in this case the trigger is the fact that the sexual abuse is not only the reason that I can't discuss my childhood but also he threatened to kill me if I did, which makes me afraid to talk about it.

My life outside of therapy continues and, on the whole, I function well. Sometime ago Beth found a dog in Finsbury Park. She had been abandoned and was a very mangy, skinny but affectionate Border Collie. Beth nursed her back to health and Poppy, the dog, became pregnant. Beth asks if Clare and I want a pup. We are adamant that we don't. Whilst at work one evening, I am working with a client in his flat. He has the T.V. on and I suddenly see Beth on animal hospital. I ask the client to turn up the T.V. and call for my colleague to join me. All three of us watch Beth talking to Rolf Harris about the scan, which has just been carried out on her dog. Rolf Harris says, "There are seven puppies. Will you manage to find homes for them all?"
Beth replies, "Oh yes, my friend will have one, parents of my daughter's friends will have one each and my mum will have one."
I look at Jan, my colleague, and say, "It's the first I have heard of it."
When the puppies are about a week old Clare and I visit Beth. Before we leave home, I say to Clare, "You must not let me be persuaded to say that I will have a puppy."
We arrive at Beth's and can't resist picking up a puppy. This little ball of fluff licks my ear as I hold her on my chest. I look at Clare and we both nod at the same time and say

'yes' to taking this puppy. We call her Misty and five weeks later she travels in a cat box to our home, crying all the way.

Right from the very beginning, this puppy steals our hearts and quickly becomes an important part of our family. She is such a pleasure and a joy. She was the one in the litter who most liked people and it shows in her very affectionate nature. Clare and I agree that Misty is the best decision we have ever forced on us.

I begin observing a baby and her family for a year. The baby is just a few weeks old when I start. I find it fascinating as I watch this little person's personality develop. I also watch the family dynamics change because they have a new baby in the home. The baby's big brother also has to adjust to not being the only child and not being the baby of the family. It takes all of them some time to adjust. Watching the baby's development in such a focused way makes me aware of how vital it is that the mother relates to her baby's wants and needs and learns how her baby communicates those needs to her. The mother is also aware that her four and a half year old son desires to be her only baby. If left unattended, the little boy will pinch and bite his new baby sister. When she is feeding at her mother's breast, the little boy tries to push his baby sister off of his mother's lap to sit there himself. Sometimes his mother gives in to him and puts the baby down and gives him a cuddle. As his baby sister gets bigger, her eyes follow her big brother as he plays in the same room. They start to relate with one another in a playful way. As their eyes meet the baby girl beams a big smile at her brother and he begins to take more of an interest in her rather than pushing her away from their mother.

Seeing a good mother makes me aware of all that I missed and I am sad at this loss.

CHAPTER TWELVE
I FIND INFORMATION ABOUT MY PAST

For many years I have tried to find out about my early childhood. As a teenager, I had asked officials if they had any information on my father. Nothing was ever forthcoming. As I got older, I asked Islington Social Services if they had any official written information about the years that I was in care. The answer was always no.

In 1997 Clare suggests that I try again. I am not sure which borough I was born in, Islington or Hackney. I know that I was born in the Finsbury Park area but one part of Finsbury Park is in Islington, the other is in Hackney. I write to the London borough of Hackney. I have written to them before with no success but I think they are worth trying again. As I work for Islington Social Services, I go to see the person who is in charge of the children and families section in Islington. I wait for two or three months but there isn't any reply from either of the boroughs.

At work one day a phone call comes through for me. It is from a social worker that is working for the London Metropolitan Archives. She tells me, "Ms Smart, I have received a letter from Hackney Social Services stating that you have been trying to locate your file." I am intrigued to know where this is going. She goes on to say, "We have a file on your family and you can make an appointment to come and look through it."

I make an appointment to meet with her at the London Metropolitan Archives in two weeks time.

Two weeks later I leave work early and Clare meets me at the tube station. We make the rest of the journey together. When we arrive at the London Metropolitan Archives, which reminds me of a library because it is so quiet, a middle-aged woman, who introduces herself as the social worker who spoke to me on the phone, meets us. She tells me that the files that are kept in this building have just become open files. I ask, "What does that mean?"

She says, "Until 1997 all these files that are about the children that have been in care were closed files and members of the public, including the people who they are about, were not allowed to see them."

I think to myself, "So, every time that I inquired whether there was any information about me and was told that there was none it had been a lie. For all those years, all those officials had lied to me."

The social worker leaves the room to fetch my file. She returns with a brown manila file that has a white ribbon tied around it. She sits down and opens the file. She partly covers the file and takes out sheets of paper and places them face down on the table. She tells me in a kindly voice, "These pieces of paper are about your brothers and there are medical reports etcetera."

She looks at me with a soft gentle look and says, "I am sorry, but you are not allowed to see them."

The social worker explains that the file is in two parts. She says, "The 'Officers Report' section is the record of the various child welfare officer's contacts with your family. The other section contains reports and memos between May 1950 and August 1956."

The first letter that I read is a report from the area children's officer.

Dear Miss Rulings,

Here is the report on the Smart family as I promised you on the telephone this morning.
There are three children: Joe 12/10/45, Dennis 10/4/47 and Pamela 5/11/49.

Mr Smart has apparently been in and out of prison throughout his married life and during his spells at home has been extremely violent and cruel, knocking his wife about, even when she was pregnant.
The other tenants in the house are terrified of him and lock their doors when he is at home.
Burglary seems to be one of his offences, and he apparently rifled all the gas meters in the house prior to his last sentence. I am not sure whether he leads an immoral life in any other direction as I only have the report of his sister-in-law but she thinks that he does consort with other women!

Clare and I manage a smile because clearly the language used in these reports is dated. We read on.

The actual living premises are very poor, most of the furniture having been broken up from time to time by Mr Smart. There are 3 rooms, including one bedroom, one kitchen/living room and the third room is too damp to use. These are all on the ground floor.
The circumstances leading up to the present crisis are these. During the last confinement Mrs Smart had such a terrible time with her husband that she decided to divorce him. He actually kept her walking the streets when she was in labour, as the police were looking for him. He has been in prison since the birth of the baby and is due out in 6 months time. Apparently he has been sending her threatening messages and the object, which has obsessed her mind, was to get the children away to a place of safety. This apparently unhinged her mind.
Mrs Smart's sister is really not in a position to continue to care for these children, although she has done every thing possible to help in every way.
I hope this report will be of help to you in dealing with this case.

Health Visitor

My mother was admitted to Brentwood mental hospital at this time.
The social worker shows me the 'Officers Report' section of the file. The first date that was entered was:

12/5/50 - Mrs Edith phoned Mrs Smart's sister - a case for taking children into care.
16/5/50 - From the report received from the Health visitor, I consider that we should take the 3 children into care if vacancies are available. If not, then I think this matter should be discussed with the sister to ascertain whether accommodation can be made available and also whether objections to taking the children are financial.
19/5/50 - Vacancy at Ladywell for Pamela.
20/5/50 - Admitted today (Pamela).
9/6/50 - Mrs Smart's sister telephoned to ask whether we could take the other two children into care. She cannot continue to look after them. The father will be home soon. She fears that he will harm them.
9/6/50 - Notified that children were taken from Day Nursery to Lamorbey children's home.

I stop looking through the officer's report from time to time as different people have written it by hand and most of the report is extremely difficult to read. I ask the social worker, "Where is Ladywell nursery, the nursery that I had been taken to at six months old? What type of nursery would it be?"
She tells me in a soft voice, "Ladywell Nursery was in the borough of Lewisham."
She shows me another piece of paper, which reads: "Baby Smart was collected and taken to Ladywell Nursery." I feel so sad and tears run down my cheeks as I realise that I

have always had a secret fantasy that I had stayed with one of my mother's sisters until I was much older, before being sent to a residential Nursery.

I am given time to get myself together before continuing. She says, "You would have been taken by car across London from Hackney to Lewisham."

Her voice drifts away as I imagine that I am like a package or a parcel being collected and dumped in this strange place. Her voice comes into focus, "Ladywell Nursery was an old workhouse and it would have housed small children and elderly people although they would have been in separate parts of the building. Ladywell Nursery was a day nursery and a place where babies stayed for a short period of time, perhaps while their mum was in hospital having another child."

Workhouse? Nothing makes any sense. I hate feeling this anger and hatred. It eats me up and makes me feel so bad inside. I hang my head down as I find it difficult to absorb all of this. I am asked if I am all right. Clare puts her arm around my shoulder as the social worker continues, "It would have been unusual for any baby to stay there for twenty six months."

She shows me several documents, "These are requests for you to be 'boarded out', and this was the term used for fostering. There were many requests for 'boarding out' during the time that you were at Ladywell. About every two months, the Matron at Ladywell sent the Welfare Officer a request for you to be 'boarded out' and the Welfare Officer replied to the matron that it was not in the best interests of your mother, who was mentally unstable and threatened, to take you out of care if you were 'boarded out'."

From the information that I piece together from the Officers Report, which was like a diary of significant events, my mother stopped visiting me at Ladywell Nursery after a few weeks because she found it too distressing, The report says that she was distressed by the fact that her baby looked away from her and no longer recognised her.

I stayed at Ladywell Nursery for twenty-six months before being transferred to Lamorbey children's home, which I knew as the Hollies children home in Sidcup Kent.

Nanny Donnelly had told me that at this time I was very ill and that she had fought for me to be placed with my brothers at the Hollies.

Whilst going through all the loose-leaf paper work, which makes up my file, I come across two other significant pieces of information. The first was one of the entries in the Officers Report. It seems that the Welfare Officer was having difficulties in getting to see my mother. She had been discharged from the hospital but was not at her house or at her mother's house.

31/4/51 - I visited at 7pm. I was told that Mrs Smart did not reside there. The informant was a very foreign woman who spoke little English. I insisted that Mrs Smart rented the ground floor but on entering I found the place empty. However, her brother, whom I had previously interviewed, was there and he explained that the house had been sold and the new owner has arranged for Mrs Smart to rent only two rooms on the second floor. The brother, on request of the owner, was completing the decoration on the ground floor and the owner was decorating the new accommodation. Mr Samuels said his sister would not be home until tomorrow as she was working until 6.55pm and, until the new tenants moved in, she was sleeping at a friend's house. I saw her rooms. They are smaller than the other rooms she was renting and would not be much use if she had all three children with her. For the time being the woman's temporary address is: 15, Durham Road N. 4 and she is paying 25/- per week rent. Her brother further said that every time Mrs Smart visited Pamela she had a further outburst of hysteria and cried for days on returning home and kept threatening to remove her from the nursery.

I look at Clare in disbelief. The man in the Officers Report that has been identified as my mother's brother must have been Uncle Harry. My mother never had a brother who was close to her or would have helped her and 15 Durham Road was Nanny Donnelly's address. She was living with Uncle Harry and his mother and he was passing himself off as her brother.

An entry for 29/5/51 catches my attention. How easily the authorities were fobbed off! My mother says that she has to have hospital treatment for six months and the Welfare Officer does not contact her for another six months although there continue to be recommendations for me to be "boarded out". It seems that the authorities took everything that my mother and her family told them at face value. They were told that my father was violent and hit my mother and that he was in prison. I can't see that there was any attempt to find out if this was true. My mother lived with Uncle Harry and his mother. The authorities never checked out this address. She passed Uncle Harry off as her brother but they never questioned his identity.

29/5/51 - A further shocking discovery I made was a letter supposedly written by my mother but it was written in Uncle Harry's handwriting. Suddenly seeing his handwriting has brought uncle Harry into the room. I can feel myself hyperventilating. I feel afraid and it takes a while before I can read the letter.
It makes me feel so angry that they hadn't picked up on this. His handwriting was very clearly different from my mother's. I read the letter that he has written and I show it to Clare. I say, "What a creep. It's such a grovelling letter."
The letter read as follows:

Wednesday, April 23rd 1952

Dear Miss Greenwood,

I hope you will forgive me troubling you, but I feel that I would be very much more settled if, when the appropriate time arrives, you would consider sending my baby, Pamela, to the same children's home as Joe and Dennis, as they are always asking about her.
I visited Joe and Dennis every visiting time but, unfortunately, I have not visited Pamela as often as I should have liked. Every time I have seen her, it has taken weeks for me to get over the emotional strain, so I have been forced by this to curtail my visits. I believe if they were together, it would ease the pain of separation a little.
I know I am a great source of expense to the L.C.C. and I cannot think of words to express my grateful and heartfelt thanks. I am so sorry to be such a burden to you and your department, so if it is possible to arrange this matter, I would be so pleased.
Thank you so much for this letter. Mrs Greenwood, I am again so sorry to be such a nuisance.

Yours most sincerely

Mrs Smart

Clearly there was a lot of manipulation going on and I suspect that Uncle Harry led my mother. The pattern is so similar to what happened in my childhood when I returned home.
I was transferred to the Hollies on the 7th of July 1952.
The next entry in the report isn't made until 13/6/55, three years later.

Phoned Miss Wheeler, Welfare Officer, re Mrs Smart meeting. Mrs Smart says that she visited once a month during March, April and May. She always looks prosperous and flourishing. Mrs Wheeler feels that Mrs Smart is very casual as when Joe was in trouble. Mrs Wheeler saw Joe as wanting to go home with his mother. The family does not seem to be doing anything differently. Mrs Wheeler agrees that Mrs Smart does not want to accept the responsibility after all these years.

In a report of 18/8/1955 it states:

I told her that we were concerned about Joe's behaviour lately and that we felt that his conduct resulted from his sense of insecurity and separation from her. I pointed out that, if we were to avert a repetition of his behaviour, she should have him home.
Mrs Smart became rather belligerent at this stage and thought that I should be saying all of this to her husband who is now out of prison. I impressed upon her the importance of giving the matter some serious thought. I further stated that the children had been in care for more than six years and that this was a large portion out of a child's life.
She appeared to be in good health, was very well dressed and stated that she was in full employment.

There were numerous entries detailing my mother's dealings with the welfare officer, requests for the children to live at home and money owed by her to the local authority. She must have been obliged to make a small contribution. There was quite a lot of manipulation to get better housing and furnishings before she would consent to have the children home.

12/3/56 - Mrs Smart now says she will have Joe and Dennis home as soon as she is re-housed.
18/8/56 - Mrs Smart is at her new home and she says that she will collect the 3 children on Sunday 2/9/56.

I find a note in the file saying that the family should be visited once a month and the situation should be monitored. No visits by the authorities are ever made. This shocks me as my mother had a history of mental illness and obviously didn't want us home. At this point the file was closed.

I made arrangements with the Social Worker at the London Metropolitan Archives for copies of the papers that I have seen to be photocopied and sent to my home. As I leave this huge building, I think about all the children's stories that are stored in this mausoleum, being closely guarded like precious gems. The children whose history is kept here are never going to know about themselves or their past, nor is the world. It is as if they are being kept secret and out of sight, just as we were as children. I can see Michael's face, a boy who was a bit older than me. He was my friend when we were in the same house together at the Hollies. I can picture his face and as he turns to look at me. I can see the lifelessness in his eyes and how this reflects my own dead and destroyed soul at the time before I started therapy.

Looking through the file informs me and confirms how manipulative my mother was. I hadn't imagined it. I am stunned by the blatant lies that were told about Uncle Harry being my mother's brother and it reminds me of what we now know about paedophiles, how they get involved with a family with the sole intention of abusing a child. I also feel anger about how inept the authorities were. They knew that my mother had mental health issues and yet they allowed us to remain in care for almost seven years and then let us return home with no follow-ups. During the years of abuse, whilst living at home with my mother and Uncle Harry, none of this information was given to the local school, G.P. or any other professional that was responsible for my well-being. Instead, the information was carefully stored away and guarded, thus ensuring that no one, including myself, could ever find out where it was.

There are so many gaps in the Welfare Officers record and sadly there are no records of my day-to-day life at Ladywell Nursery or the Hollies children's home. No photographs, no family who can tell me what I was like as a child. I feel that I have no history. I decide to contact the borough of Lewisham. That is the borough in which Ladywell Nursery was situated. They write back saying that there was no record of me being in the care of Lewisham. I telephone the person that has written to me. She suggests that maybe my records had been sent to the London borough of Bexley when I was transferred to the Hollies. I try Bexley local authority. They tell me that my file has probably been given back to the borough of Hackney when I went to live with my mother. I have gone a full circle. I am back to Hackney social services, which also deny any responsibility.
I write to Hackney Social Services. In my letter I write, "It is my understanding that records of children in care have to be kept for seventy-five years before they can be destroyed."
I never receive a reply. I go to see my local MP. She writes to all three boroughs concerned. All three boroughs deny any knowledge or responsibility. Neither Ladywell Nursery or The Hollies exist any longer: the Hollies closed down in the early eighties and Bexley social services tell me that they have no idea where all the files went after the children's home closed down. What's worse is that no one

cares what happened to all those files that hold so many stories of all the children that were placed in their care.

I often feel that the story about my roots is not one that people want to hear. When I am with a group of friends and they are talking about their families, their elderly mother, aunty or some other member of their extended family, I feel excluded. If they talk about a place or an event that happened to them when they were growing up, I again feel excluded. The discussion suddenly goes silent if I reveal even a minor part of my story. I sense people backing away. My friends look embarrassed and they don't know what to say. I tell Sue how I have felt at different times when this happened to me. She thinks that when I do not talk about that part of my life, I also keep the secret. I collude in a similar way to all those people who colluded, with a wall of silence, throughout the years that I was growing up.

CHAPTER THIRTEEN
THERAPY WITH SUE CONTINUES

The following weekend I am walking in our local park with Clare. I see small children in their pushchairs with their parents and I see other little family groups, where the children are playing on their bikes or skates. I feel a huge rage. I hate these perfect families that seem to have everything. I think of myself being collected like a parcel and dumped in that strange place at six months old. I tell Sue about the anger that I feel. I say, "I bet I was never taken out, let alone taken out to a park. Was I imprisoned in that place?"

I am back there. "I can see the rows of cots and see parents who have come to collect their children at the end of the day. I hate them. Why have they been chosen and not me? Am I bad? I feel bad. I feel so very bad and maybe that's why I am dumped. A workhouse. How could they dump me in a workhouse? Nothing makes any sense. I hate feeling this anger and hatred. It eats me up and makes me feel so bad inside."

I tell Sue, "I feel this at times when I am left alone or feel abandoned like when you go away on holidays and when there is a break in therapy. It feels like it's the end of the world."

I continue with my course and for the most part I enjoy it. I find many aspects of my training fascinating and stimulating. When one of the seminar leaders uses children's storybooks as a tool for looking at psychological aspects of the characters and the situations described in the stories, I feel stupid and at a disadvantage because I do not know the stories and the other students do. I never had any stories read to me and when my own children were young I could not read well enough to read stories to them. However, in the event, I find that it is not a disadvantage. Indeed, perhaps I look at the stories with fresh eyes. One of the stories we use is 'The Little Prince' who visits different worlds. On each world is a person or animated objects, e.g. a flower. Characters have different emotional disorders or pathologies. Although the children reading the stories might have thought that they were strange, they would not have recognised that they were suffering from a mental disorder. Because I did not know the story, I did not hold any previous ideas about it and was clearly able to see what the tutor was looking for.

It's Saturday afternoon and Clare and I go to visit a friend who lives in the area of Denmark Hill. To get there we have to drive through Cold Harbour Lane, in Brixton. Cold Harbour Lane is a well-known red light district. As we drive through there, I start to feel nervous. I am twitchy and alarm bells start to ring in my head. I think to myself 'danger, danger,' I don't like this place. I say to Clare, "Hurry up, speed up. I don't want to get caught up at the lights. I must get out of this area." Clare reassures me that we will be all right. She says, "It's day time, there is no need to panic; red light districts mainly operate at night."

My anxiety has subsided by the time we have arrived at my friend's house. We have some lunch and then decide to take our dog for a walk. We walk to a small green near my friend's flat. I am in a strange area, which seems run down. I begin to feel very cold and frightened. I am shivering and I have pains all over my body. I say to Clare, "Can we go back to Sally's flat? I don't like it here and I am freezing cold." We walk back to Sally's flat, but I still feel icy cold and very anxious. I can't shake this feeling off. It only goes when I am safely back in my own home.

At therapy I describe my experience to Sue. Sue encourages me to talk through the images. I start by telling her about my visit to my friend's house. Then, like a moving picture on a cinema screen, lots of different images of different places at different times in my childhood run through my mind. It is as if I am watching a fruit machine and waiting for the different symbols to stop flashing past and settle on to one memory. The images slow down, then my mind settles on one picture. The more I try to find the words for what I am seeing, the more difficult I find it. I feel so fragmented as the past and the present blur into one. I let the blurring continue and I don't fight against it, instead I allow the past and the present to intermingle.

I say, "Sue, I can see 'her'. 'She' has run away from home, 'she' is lying on the grass near the reservoir, near to that flat.
I am so cold. I feel scared. I hate them and they hate me. It's dark and I have been here all night. I'm so cold.
'She' walks the streets until the underground opens, then 'she' gets on to the tube and runs from carriage to carriage, hoping that she will fall between the doors onto the track.
'She' is back on the streets again. Her mother is there and asks 'her': Is it true? Is he touching you? 'Her' mother says that she will protect 'her' but she doesn't. She says that she has to stay with him. 'Her' mother tells 'her' not to tell because she can not live without him."

The scene changes: 'She' is sleeping rough. 'She' is in the red light district. It's sleazy but she doesn't care. All those men. All those men. 'She' is scared."
Sue says, "She is you."
"My head is spinning, Sue".
Sue says, "Just let your head spin, go with it. I'm here."

I hold my head to stop it from spinning. The room is spinning and I feel ill.

Sue gently puts her hand on my head and I feel held.

I say, "I'm scared. I am in a strange place. I am blindfolded. Those men took me to a strange place. They gave me drugs, did things to me and then dumped me."

Sue asks, "What things did they do to you?"

I can't find the words to describe that memory. I am crying and saying, "I am sorry, I am so sorry. Please don't hate me."

Sue waits, then puts a hand on my back and says, "It's O.K., Pam."

The words come tumbling out. "Sue, all these men have sex with me, one after the other. I feel so dirty and ashamed."

For the rest of the session we piece together how what I was feeling when visiting my friend linked to this memory of being raped and my shame about it. I can recall with Sue lots of other occasions when I am out and I suddenly do not feel safe. Sue says, "I can imagine that you are always aware of not feeling safe. The anxiety of feeling unsafe is always there with you, like a backdrop to your life waiting to emerge."

I think the memory of meeting my mother at the underground station was a screen memory that covered the memory of the gang rape.

At another therapy session I tell Sue about certain foods that I cannot eat. I explain that whilst I was on a training workshop with MIND this issue came up. People were talking about different foods that they liked and didn't like. When it came to my turn I gave a list of foods that I hated. Even thinking about them made me feel sick. I told them that all these foods were related to Uncle Harry. I told Sue how I felt that I had been hit over the head with a brick when the course leader interpreted my dislike of these

foods and how it was linked with Uncle Harry as, "You don't want him inside you."
I have never thought of that before. Sue asks me what the foods were and I list them off. Custard, rice pudding, custard cream biscuits, apple pie, apples, tea, milk and numerous other foods and drinks that make me feel sick. There are certain smells that also reminded me of him. Sue asked me if I want to bring in one of the foods to my next session.

I choose the two foods that I hate the most, rice with custard. I bring a little pot in with me. Once we enter the consulting room, I take the pot of Muller rice out of my bag and place it on the floor next to me. Sue holds the pot in front of me and gets me to look at it.
My reaction is, "Ugh, no, I don't like it."
I try to push it away from my face. Sue encourages me to look at it and says, "Let whatever feelings or thoughts that come into your head just come."
I look at this tub of rice with custard and I freeze. I feel paralysed and just stare at it.
Sue says, "I want you to try and put some on your lips."
As I do so, I heave. I can feel my mouth filling up with saliva. I frantically wipe it off my lips with the back of my hand saying, "No, I don't like this. I really do not like this."
I try to spit it out. I keep spitting into a hanky and I begin to heave. Then I begin to choke. I say, "I can't get this stuff out of my mouth and I lay on the floor trying to will the taste to go away. "Please go away," I say.
I am choking, heaving and trying to get the taste out of my mouth. There is a smell of sex and that makes me heave. I retch and a choking sensation makes me panic. I think that it is the end. I can't breathe.

Sue put an arm around me and gently brings my mind back into the present. Sue says, "I noticed that the whole area around your mouth had turned white and your face was flushed and very red."

I had been reliving an experience of oral sex. I ask Sue in a shaky voice, "Please, can you take that away?" I point at the tub of Muller rice. "It's still making me feel sick."

Sue takes it out of the room and throws it away. She brings me back a glass of water to take the taste away.

Even until this day, I do not like these foods. They still make me feel sick. We decide that, as these foods are not essential in my life, we will not pursue my hatred for them any further.

The psychotherapy that Sue uses with me is mainly primal psychotherapy, which is a mixture of primal therapy and ordinary psychotherapy with interpretations, transference and counter transference and attachment theories together with Kleinian theories. There is no end to the things that keep coming up in therapy. There are never any silences or hesitations. There are, however, changes in myself. I have become less angry and panicky about situations that remind me of my past. I become more aware and able to identify irrational feelings. With Sue's help, I can see where they came from and where they belong in my past.

On the whole, Sue is very gentle with me, although there are times when she sounds exasperated. I occasionally adamantly hold on to a pathological idea, an idea that is usually crazy, often involving envy. When this happens Sue says, "Pam, you are losing the plot and we are not going there!"

I protest and tell her that she just doesn't understand how unfair life has been to me. But as therapy has developed, I come to understand that if I persist with these thoughts and feelings I feel much worse about myself.

The split has slowly come together. I am now able to talk about my child self as me. I no longer hate that part of me.

I continue to work hard both at work and with my psychotherapy course. My son Jay gets married and a few months later his wife gives birth to a baby daughter. Amy is lovely and a very bright baby.

Jay and his family move to a small village in Kent. Clare and I are not able to be as involved with Jay's baby as we are with Beth and her daughter because Jay lives so far away from us. We do, however, visit them and they regularly visit us.

CHAPTER FOURTEEN
MY PAST CATCHES UP WITH ME PHYSICALLY

Islington Social Services have decided to restructure my post and amalgamate it with the deputy's post, which will create one new post. If I take up the new post, I will earn less money and I will have more work. I take the option of early retirement.

I leave in the April of 2000. I am concentrating on my course, working with psychotherapy training clients and attending the gym, in an attempt to get myself physically fit. Working full time and training as a psychotherapist left little time for me to go to the gym or to go swimming. I had forgotten how much I enjoy physical activities. I have always been very sporty, especially when I was younger.

Five months have past since leaving Islington Social Services. A friend tells me that Lambeth College is looking for someone to teach counselling skills as a visiting tutor. I meet with the head of department and, after some formalities, I start teaching for three teaching sessions a week at the beginning of the autumn term. Soon I am interviewed and promoted to a permanent post as a lecturer, teaching counselling to mature students. I enjoy this work. It is new to me, so very different from my work with Islington. The students come from diverse cultures and backgrounds and most are very keen to learn. A lot of them are already in employment and want to enhance their communication skills when working with people or they want to change careers. Some students have been out of employment for one reason or another, perhaps having started a family and there are two or three students who have physical disabilities.

******

It's Saturday and I'm on a weekend training seminar for my course. We watch two videos. I find that both of them fed back into my past and I find them upsetting on both occasions. The first video that we watch is a training documentary made by the Robertson's, who researched the effects on children who have been separated from their parents. It was set in the early fifties and was about a young toddler who had been in residential care whilst his mother went into hospital to have a new baby. The film showed in detail how distressed the little boy became in the new, strange environment where he had been left. The little boy, 'John', was left in residential care for about a week. He didn't want to eat and clung to members of staff until they picked him up. All the other children in the film had been left in care permanently. These little children grabbed at the food on the table, took food from other children's bowls and grabbed attention from the staff when and if they could. I never saw any of the other children cry for attention. They screamed when another child hit them and any screaming or yelling was short lived. I stopped watching John in the film as my attention was focused on a little girl about two and a half years old. She had blond curly hair and when she grabbed for food or the other children's toys and couldn't get them, she hit the other kids. John couldn't compete with the other children and cried until he was picked up. The member of staff in the film was shown carrying him around with her wherever she went. The little blond girl attempted to push John off her lap and she was gently pushed away. When the video had finished the room was silent. It was an upsetting video to watch. The first student who spoke said that she could identify with John and that the other children had never had parents, so they didn't become upset because they couldn't miss what they had never had. I had felt upset during the film and now I feel furious. I challenge the student who made this statement and tell her that she is wrong, "Those children probably craved closeness with the adult carers as much as John. I could identify with the other children who had been in care for a long time."

The seminar leader asks me if there was any child in particular with whom I identified and I tell her that I identified with the little blond girl. The seminar leader agrees with me that, although the film had been made to show how distressed a small child becomes when the attachment with his parents or carers is broken even for a short time, John in fact was making demands and getting time and attention from the staff but the other children who were living at the nursery got even less attention while John was there. John was going to return to a caring family. The other children were going to be left and the damage to them would be far greater than the damage that was done to John as a result of what he experienced.

The other video is about a woman in her forties who has just come out of a long stay psychiatric hospital. She had been in hospital since she was a teenager and had originally been admitted because she was dysfunctional. She had been brought up in a poor run down area and with a family who were very disturbed. Over the years she had been given different medication and Electro-Convulsive Therapy (E.C.T.). She was given this treatment and kept in hospital for such a long time because she self harmed and had attempted suicide on several occasions. She had now left hospital after spending over twenty years there.

I find it shocking that no one had been there to help this disturbed teenager who consequently spent her life as a young woman in an institution. I feel that this could have been avoided. I thought about myself at that age and how the psychiatrist who was treating me told the juvenile magistrate that I should be sent to a special hospital. It was only while I was in therapy with Helle that I realised what this might have meant for me. Helle asked me, "What do you think the psychiatrist meant when he said special hospital?"

I had said that I did not know. Helle said that she thought that I had a guardian angel looking after me because she thought they meant Broadmoor or Rampton.

I left the room where the training was taking place, took myself to a private space and wept for that woman and for my teenage self.

I took both of these experiences to therapy. I talk about the film of John in the residential children's home. I begin to go back into my own past. I close my eyes.

Sue asks me, "What is happening, Pam?"

I say, "They have shut me in a room. I have been bad. I feel bad."

Sue says, "You feel bad."

I stretch my arms up waiting to be picked up. Sue is silent. I search for her with my hands in a grasping movement. The room is quiet and I feel so alone. Sue has left me alone. A wave of panic sweeps over me and the ground is moving, the walls split. I lay very still. I feel paralysed.

Sue says, "What is happening? Try to find some words."

I say, "I'm scared. I've been bad. I might be hit. I must lie down and be quiet and stay still. I love you, Sue. I love you and I won't be bad."

When Sue and I talked about this afterwards she thought that it might relate to the time when I was placed in the nursery at six months old.

Then I begin to feel that I am an older child, maybe a toddler and maybe I have been put into another room because I had been bad. Perhaps I have hit the other children. In the regression, I search for someone to pick me up. My arms are extended. A face appears in my mind's eye and feelings of excitement rush through me.

Sue represents the face of the nurse or carer. Sue thinks this face could have been my wish for a mother.

I discovered with Sue that the words "I love you" are used by me as a defence to make me feel better and block out unpleasant and unwanted feelings. The words "I love you" bring on the feelings attached to the mother in the sky. This makes me feel loveable, normal and not disintegrated, which is the feeling I most fear.

This defence is what has undoubtedly enabled me to survive emotionally, and that is why it has been the most difficult defence to dismantle in therapy. For me to let go of this, I had to allow myself to feel very alone, abandoned and vulnerable. It was only when I was able to let go of this defence that I could begin to mourn my lost childhood, to face the reality and grieve for what I did not have.

In another session I recall with Sue standing at the gate of the children's home watching and waiting for a mother to come for me and take me away. I have always been aware that children might be adopted although I did not realise until I gained possession of my file that adoption had never been an option because my mother and uncle Harry refused to allow it, presumably each having their own agenda as to why.

Screen memories are coming up in therapy, that is, memories that in themselves are not traumatic but which serve to mask traumatic memories. Though not traumatic, they are persistent.

In my mind I go back to a time when I was a small child sitting under nanny Donnelly's table, rocking myself backwards and forwards. My mother, uncle Harry and nanny Donnelly are in the room and in my head I can hear the rhyme, "See you later alligator, in a while crocodile".

As this memory comes up, I feel scared but I don't know why. I can't make out why the boys are not there. I tell Sue,

"I'm scared. I don't know why. I can see my mother and nanny Donnelly. Uncle Harry is in his underpants. He is always in his underpants or he sits with his trousers undone. His thing is always out. He does this at the camp. He sits down at the table and his thing comes out of his underpants."
Sue asks me, "Do you have a name for his thing?"
I put my hand out, palm facing outwards as if pushing it away. I say, "No, no name. I don't have a name."
I look away and say, "I don't want to see it."
The scene changes. I say, "I am back in that flat, he is leaning over my bed. His thing is out and I have to hide my eyes, pretend that I am asleep. I feel a pain in my back like a heavy weight on my back."
Sue gently places a hand on my back. I can feel the pressure. The pressure becomes unbearable. I shout out at the same time as sobbing. "Get off, you fucking bastard, get off of me. I don't like it. No, no, I don't like it. Get off of me, get off."
I begin to calm down. I love you, Sue. I love you. I need to feel safe. I won't be bad."

The other screen memory that comes up continually is an image of me at the children's home going to the woods. The woods are a group of trees that are at the side of the main path that leads to the big gates of the children's home. I can see myself as a small child of three or four. I tell Sue, "Sue, I feel scared. I made such a fuss and I wouldn't go home for the weekend. Joe is cross with me. He says it's my fault that Mummy hasn't come this weekend. Mummy Robins says that I am bad for making such a fuss. I am all alone and I go into the woods to play with the trees. The song "Teddy bear's picnic" is in my head. I can hear the words. The trees are the teddy bears and I feed them. I feel sad. Those deep crying pains are in my tummy. I love you, Sue. I love you."

These images come and go in my therapy sessions. I also find that they come up in my mind when I am not at therapy.

Sue tells me about a new course that she has been on. It is called E.M.D.R, which stands for Eye Movement Desensitisation and Reprocessing. Sue explains that E.M.D.R. can be a helpful way to help someone who has been traumatised, where the trauma has not been worked through. It consists of stimulating each side of the brain alternately by eye movement or tapping each hand or each foot alternately, or in each ear alternately by audible tones. The patient initially holds in their mind an image representing the trauma and a negative statement as to how they feel as a result of the trauma. The negative feelings reduce as the treatment progresses. At the end of the treatment a positive statement as to how the patient would like to feel is introduced and, by means of the therapy, installed.

Sue uses this with me a few times. It brings up a large amount of detail about the trauma. We are still focussing on issues that have been looked at before, only this time in more detail and from a different aspect. The only unhelpful thing that I find when Sue uses this method is I tend to get left with feelings that then need to be discharged later.

The familiar image of me sitting under Nanny Donnelly's table comes up again. My negative feeling about myself is that I feel helpless. Sue taps my feet alternately. The image in my head is frozen. I can see everything so clearly. I can't see myself under the table but I can see Nanny Donnelly standing at the kitchen sink, my mother is just standing there and uncle Harry has just entered the room in his underclothes. I think he has arrived home from work and is changing out of his work clothes. The rhyme

'See you later alligator, in a while crocodile' slips in and out of my mind. The scene changes, I can see in detail the wallpaper in the passageway: brown wallpaper and brown paintwork. I say to Sue, "I'm scared, Sue. I love you, I love you."

Sue says, "It's Ok, Pam. Tell me what is happening and, if at any time you find it too much, we can stop."

I say, "I'm small. I can see me and I'm small. I am in the passageway and my mother is walking behind me. She is guiding me towards his bedroom door. She opens the door and gently pushes me inside the room. He is in bed and he is beckoning me to go to him. I am filled with panic as I realise that my mother has gone. She has left me alone in his bedroom. I see myself walking towards his bed. Uncle Harry pulls me up on to his bed. He covers me with his bedclothes. Ah ah, he is rubbing up against me. No, no, the room is spinning around. Sue, I don't like it. My head hurts, I can't breathe. Sue, I'm wet. I have wet myself. He throws me off of his bed and shouts to my mother, "The filthy little bitch has wet herself. Get her cleaned up."

Sue brings my mind back into the room. I ask her, "Will you hold my hand?"

Sue sits beside me and lets me hold her hand. We talk about what came up. I cannot believe it had happened. I find it shattering. My mother took me to his room, she cleaned me, and what was it she cleaned off of me? Had I wet myself or was it semen?

I am perplexed about the fact that my brothers are not there. I think back to the time when we went home from the children's home at the weekend. I try to work it out. Where were my brothers? I say to Sue, "I think that they stayed with my Aunty Rachel. They stayed with Aunty Rachel and her family and I stayed with my mother and uncle Harry at Nanny Donnelly's home. There was not enough room for my brothers to stay there as well. No doubt he had his reasons why the boys were not there anyway."

After this session and for several weeks I go over this with Clare. Did my mother know? Did nanny Donnelly know? They must have.

Over the next few weeks Sue and I work through a lot of the feelings that this memory has brought up. The image of sitting under the table also becomes clearer. There was a perverse sexual game being carried out by uncle Harry. His penis was the crocodile and he said the rhyme as he played with himself. I come to an acceptance that my mother must have been aware of what was going on. Nanny Donnelly must have also had some awareness of what was happening although this is something that I find very painful to think of. I tell Sue about my memories of not wanting to leave the children's home with my mother and uncle Harry. I talk to her about my confusion as pieces of memory come together. I constantly ask, "Am I right? Did this really happen? Did it happen then?"

Sue explains that what I remember and feel doesn't have to stand up in a court of law and that what is important is how I feel about myself now, although, given the factual evidence about my history, she thinks that it did happen.

I tell Sue how I remember in more detail about my mother complaining about Mummy Robins at the children's home. My mother says to Mummy Robins, "You spoil her. That's why she won't come home. The housemother who looked after Joe and Dennis advised my mother to have me transferred to her house. I recall her saying, "You get her moved to my house and I will knock it out of her."

I tell Sue that I think that I tried to tell Mummy Robins about what went on when I went home with my mother and uncle Harry. My mother made sure that no further questions were asked. I wonder if this was why Mummy Robins distanced herself from me. Perhaps she feared losing her job. That is one of the many things I will never know.

I see Sue for therapy on Wednesday mornings and go to work at Lambeth College straight from therapy. The tube journey takes about an hour and I arrive for work about half an hour before I am due to teach a group of students. There are times when I feel dreadful, the thoughts and feelings from my therapy session are still so alive. Sometimes a short phone call to Sue makes me feel better, at other times I just have to put my feelings to one side until I have finished work. Once I get home from work I can tell Clare about what has come up in the session with Sue and Clare supports me in the best way that she can. She doesn't push me to be happy or to put on a show. I can just be with how I feel, which is usually pretty shitty.

Images of the children's home come up in therapy regularly, particularly of the grounds, which were extensive. There is one time when I recall sitting looking out of the window. It was my birthday and I hoped that somebody special would come and visit. It must have been a weekday because nobody came. I remember often feeling alone and how I would frequently take myself to the main gate waiting and looking for somebody to visit me or want to adopt me. When no one came I played by myself in the woods. I always thought that the memory of the woods was a good memory. The trees did not let me down. They stayed. They did not disappear. When I went into the woods I went into a world of fantasy where I would be a loved and special child, wanted by a family.

I go to therapy and I tell Sue that the tune to the 'Teddy Bear's Picnic' keeps swimming around in my head and it is making me feel uneasy. Sue asks me, "Can you sing the song, Pam? If you don't know the words, perhaps you can hum the tune?"

I don't respond. Sue taps my feet as she hums the tune. I am feeling very frightened and I can hear the words in my head.

"If you go down to the woods today, you'll be sure of a big surprise.

If you go down to the woods today, you will never believe your eyes."

In my mind's eye I suddenly see leaves on the ground, brown and golden in colour, tall trees all around me. They start to swim in a circular movement and then I'm frigid with fear. I see him. "Sue, it's him, it's uncle Harry, he is here," I say in frozen shock.

Sue asks, "What is he doing?"

I say, "He is standing here. Oh no, his trousers are down. He says, "I'm the big surprise." He undresses me and is rubbing himself against me. Afterwards he says, "You tell anyone and I will cut your tongue out. Remember my big butchers knives. I will cut you into little pieces. I am petrified with terror. I know he will do it."

When Sue brings me back into the present, I feel as if I am in stunned shock. I hadn't thought that the abuse began until later although I have very clear memories of him doing the same thing at the camp. Sue and I talk about this terrifying of me being some kind of preparation so that later on I would be so petrified that when he penetrated me I would never tell.

Everything that I have seen during this session was so vivid. I say, "I love you, Sue. I love you. Will it be alright?"

I spoke to Clare afterwards. She has worked with sex offenders and she said, "It is common for paedophiles to become involved with their victims many years before they sexually abuse them fully at an age when the child is most attractive to them. They can be very patient and groom a child for years using terror tactics, threats, and emotional blackmail and blaming the child for the abuse. The child believes this and carries the guilt. It is possible that Uncle Harry planned to abuse you from very early on. He certainly showed a lot of interest in you over the early years. Pressure from him is one explanation why your mother, who did not love you, would not allow you to be adopted and took you from the children's home."

Whenever I talk or think about Uncle Harry I am convinced that he can get to me. Even from his grave, he can get to me and hurt me. There is a part of me that still believes that he knows all that I say and all that I do. Throughout my therapy I have never been able to feel or express any anger or outrage about what he did to me. I just feel an icy cold fear, the same feeling that I have when I go back in time in my mind and see him standing in the woods at the children's home; or at nanny Donnelly's house; or at the camp and in the flat that I grew up in. The same icy cold fear sweeps over me and paralyses me.
Uncle Harry destroyed so many things, he even turned a children's song into something that put terror into my heart.

****

I'm in the last year of my psychotherapy training. I attend one evening seminar a week, together with some weekends. I am already working with training clients and during the weekends we look at the work that we, as students, are doing with our training clients and we also use role-plays in order to develop our psychotherapy skills by practice. I enjoy role-plays and really find that I come into my own. I am good at them and I can take on the role of client or therapist and really throw myself into the role. The other students find it more difficult.

****

I talk with Sue about how I feel when I'm in some of the training sessions with my fellow students: "Sometimes I say nothing in the group. I say nothing because memories about being at school come up. I feel overwhelming feelings of inadequacy and I feel as if I am being excluded from the group as I did on the Social Work course. These feelings engulf me and I can't say anything. It feels as if I am an outsider and I feel so envious that they have had a far better education than I ever had. Look at the chances that they have had."

My mind goes back to my time at school. I rant as I tell Sue, "There are no books in my house. I am made to feel that I am thick by my family. I can't read or write very well and I am continually put in a position of feeling stupid in comparison with the other children at school. Teachers single me out as worthless and of low intelligence. I always feel humiliated and I am made to feel like an outsider, excluded from the group. Other children seem to have parents who love them, they ensure that they are clean and take an interest in them and their education. I hate them and I envy them because they have loving parents, whilst I yearn for a loving mother who cares about me. Throughout all my years at school, from infancy onwards, I remember feeling so desperately alone and isolated at school."

I recall a memory where I experienced how different from mine other children's lives were. I tell Sue, "On one rare occasion, I went into the home of two girls, who were sisters. They lived on my estate. They invited me into their bedroom and I was so surprised. Their bedroom was comfortable and clean, with nice covers on the beds and matching curtains at the window. I was amazed that this space could belong to them. It was pretty and their own personal possessions were kept all around their room. This told me that care had been taken by their parents to provide this space and contrasted strongly with my lack of privacy and any place that I could call mine.

The younger sister, who I knew from school, took me into the kitchen and made salad cream sandwiches, whilst an Adam Faith record was playing on the record player. The girl's father came into the house and I froze, expecting trouble, but he simply shouted 'Hello', went to sit in the lounge and read his newspaper. My friend carried on with what she was doing. This stunned me. They had so much freedom and felt that getting a sandwich for themselves was normal and no big deal."

Sue asks, "What did you have to eat at lunchtime, Pam, when you got home from school?"

I was bewildered by the question. I said, "Food, food at lunchtime? I didn't eat at lunchtime."

The room starts to spin around. I feel the icy feeling of fear taking me over, "Food was the last thing I thought about at lunchtime. My mind was taken up with what Uncle Harry would do to me when I got home and I didn't have any time for food."

I recall with Sue what it was like to live in my world back then, "Food could not be eaten without permission, and then only at meal times. The meals that we were given were plain and the only seasonings on the table were for Uncle Harry alone. Salad cream sandwiches! Unheard of!"

"If I took food from the kitchen cupboard I was regarded as a criminal, I was punished with 'Uncle Jack'. I didn't like the food they gave me. The only food that I enjoyed eating was the sweets that I stole from the sweet shop. If I was caught, then I was caned. Always on the left hand so that I could still use my right hand for schoolwork and chores around the house."

In therapy Sue helps me to work on these issues. She encourages me to mourn and grieve for the life and parenting that I have not had. She helps me to reframe the past and to see who was really to blame, to recognise the responsible adults who should have protected me and failed to do so for what they were, inadequate for the task, incompetent and cruel. She works on my self-image and helps me to own my intelligence and know that I am not stupid. Sue points out, "You could not have achieved all that you have in your career and you could not have understood the concepts used in psychotherapy or on your course if you were stupid. There is nothing that you have said to me that would indicate that you are of low intelligence and, despite all the damage that has been done to you, your personality is very strong."

Over the years I have begun to acknowledge that my will to make things change has always remained intact. I also acknowledge that I seem to have the ability to attract professional people who have wanted to help me and they have remained in touch with me long after any professional involvement was over.

Once again there is an occasion when I become upset by the material that is being presented during a weekend training seminar. One of the other students is presenting her casework to the group, reading through her process recordings, which are sexually graphic. At first I listen with interest, then I begin to feel disturbed by the content. The more I hear, the more fragmented I feel. It feels as if the sexual material is being rammed down my throat. The seminar leader must notice my discomfort, she asks me if I am O.K. and suggests to the student that we stop here. The student says that she did need to read her work with this client and get feedback. The rest of the group and myself agree that the student continues to read her process recordings but from a different place and with less sexual content, which means that she moves on to look at other therapy sessions that she has written up. The student decides to tell us about a dream that her client had told her. She starts to read from her notes and then, to my astonishment, her notes return to sexual material. I feel overwhelmed by this, which I had asked not to hear because I was feeling disintegrated and as if I had been smashed into small pieces. I feel attacked but can't say so. I leave the room in a hurry, feeling very distressed. I just feel completely blown apart. The tutor is very supportive of me.

I take this incident and my reaction back to therapy where it can be unpicked and painful memories and feelings are worked through. It reminded me of the way that Uncle Harry talked at me for hours while I was trapped in the flat that I grew up in. In this case I had been trapped in the training room and walked out.

After five long years at L.A.P.P., my training has finally finished. It is the end of a long but worthwhile journey and I have learnt so much.

As I mentioned earlier, the training group started with four students, which reduced to a group of three. There were times when I found it very difficult as there was no place to hide in such a small group, I couldn't have a bad day and opt-out and my feelings and reactions couldn't be hidden, I was there and I was seen. However, the advantage was that we got a lot of time spent on us as individuals, and I feel very privileged as the experience was so positive and we had such excellent seminar leaders.

I continue to see my training client and am required to write my final paper, which I work on for the summer recess and for several months more.

In the past, over the years, I have experienced back problems. I had had twinges in my back and had sought osteopathy. During the period of time between finishing therapy with Helle and going on holiday with her, I had real problems with my back and had osteopathy treatment at that time.

The year before my psychotherapy course finished, I suffered a back injury at the gym. This last injury to my back never seemed to heal, indeed it got worse and after two years of putting up with severe back pain and only being able to walk a short distance without having to stop and sit down, I decide to go to my doctor and ask to have an x-ray to see what is happening. The young doctor that I see suggests that I see an osteopath who was practicing at the G.P. practice. The osteopath tells me that I have something wrong with my sacroiliac joint, which is the joint that links the pelvis bone with the spine. I attend several appointments with him. He finally says that he does not think that he can do anymore for me. I see a different doctor at the G.P. practice, which Clare has recommended. He has treated her and she values his expertise and his kindness. My first appointment with him is a different experience for me. He takes time to listen. He tells me that he has been reading through my file. He says, "Your notes start from a very important day in your life."

I look at him questioningly and I feel anxious. Clare, who is with me, says, "She is over all of that," thinking that he is referring to my breakdown all those years ago. The doctor says, "The date is the sixth of September 1969."

I smile with delight and reply, "The day that Beth was born. Yes, I remember that day very well."

I am sent for an x-ray and return to the G.P. two weeks later. He tells me that there is something showing up on the x-ray and it looks like a kink in the bottom of my spine. I am referred to a specialist at St Helier Hospital and I have to wait three months before I see him. The specialist wants me to go for a scan. He tells me that there is a waiting list of three months. I wait and then have to wait a further six months before going back to see him. He tells me that there is an abnormality showing up in the lower part of my spine.

I am referred to The Atkinson Morley Hospital. By this time my back has deteriorated. I have shooting pains down the inside of my right leg and walking has become almost impossible. I go to work and to L.A.P.P. by car. Other than this, I stay at home. My leg begins to drag along the floor when I attempt to walk and I am in a lot of pain. After a six-week wait, I go for my appointment at The Atkinson Morley. The doctor puts my scan on the viewing box. Both Clare and I are shocked when we see my spine because one of the vertebrae is not in line with the others. The doctor asks me if I can remember having injured my back at any time. I tell him about being in a plaster cast when I was a child. He says, "I think that you had fractured your back at that time. That's how fractured backs were treated in those days."

He goes on to tell me that I need an operation but that there is an eight-month waiting list. As I leave Atkinson Morley hospital, my head is reeling remembering the severe beatings by Uncle Harry and my mother and being attacked by the girls outside the children's home when I went back to visit Mummy Robins. Remembering and then seeing in a clear graphic way the damage that had been done to my body was very powerful. When I arrive home I weep for the young girl who I once was.

Needing to go into hospital for an operation brings up fears about hospitals and being treated badly. All my life I have tried to avoid hospitals and doctors. My G.P. could not understand why I hadn't seen a doctor about my back far sooner than I did, given that I had been in pain over many years. The thought had never occurred to me. I only go to see a doctor if I really have to.

Sue works with me on my fears of going into hospital for an operation. My worst fear is of going under the anaesthetic. This brings up memories of being given E.C.T. against my will and the feeling of being punished and feeling powerless while in the care of the medical professionals who I felt were hostile towards me. I am sent a letter from the hospital in November 2003 telling me that there is a bed for me at the end of that month. My G.P. has prescribed some tranquillising medication to help me over the anxious period before the operation. I have my operation on the 1st of December. I needn't have worried about my treatment in hospital because I receive respect and decent professional care throughout my stay in hospital. I also have the support of Clare, my children, my friends and Sue phones me at the hospital regularly. I can talk with her about any anxieties and fears that arise. I feel held, not abandoned as I had felt all those years ago.

After surgery, I have a follow-up appointment at the hospital. There are concerns that the operation has not been successful and, after a further scan, it is decided that I will require further surgery. My spine has slipped and is trapping the nerve down the inside of my right leg, the same nerve that was trapped before. This time the consultant says that he needs to pin the spine together with Titanium screws.

I have a second operation and I spend many months being confined to my home, only going out in the car with Clare, as I cannot walk more than a few yards. The operation has not been the success that was expected and I have been told that this level of mobility will probably not change. There are times when I feel so frustrated and helpless. I feel the same trapped and hopeless feelings that I felt when I was a child. Only now, after all I have learnt about myself and knowing that I have more resources, I have the knowledge of what works for me.

CHAPTER FIFTEEN
IN THE PRESENT DAY

I know that I have to be doing something. I cannot just be. In this time of forced idleness, which is difficult for me, I take the opportunity to write my story, which is something that I have wanted to do for a while. I want to tell my story because it is a message of hope for other people with similar experiences, who have been written off as untreatable. My illness was called many different things over the years, none of which were particularly useful or descriptive of my condition. It is clear from my experiences in therapy that I disassociated and this condition is now seen as treatable by the medical profession and by psychotherapists.

Lately my therapy has dealt with my fear of looking at Sue. When I look at her I feel disintegrated and fear seeing in her eyes what I saw in the crazy eyes of my mother, both anger and rejection. I have mourned the fact that I never really had a mother, faced the reality that that lost mothering can never be replaced and I had to come to terms with what Sue's role is in reality, which is a therapist, a good kind therapist but no less a therapist.

Therapy continues but is now far less traumatic. The body of the work has been completed. I feel happier in myself and with my life. It has been a long and productive journey that has enabled me to lead an ordinary life and given me both the personal and interpersonal skills to manage my life.
In the last year Clare and I have become members of the Metropolitan Community Church, a fully inclusive church that enables us to join in a full Christian life.

To our great pleasure the government passed a law permitting Civil Partnerships to take place between same sex couples. We contact the register office in Worthing, registering our intent on the first legal day, 5th December 2005, and we book our Civil Partnership for the 24th December 2005. We have a wonderful day supported by our relatives and friends. The registry office ceremony is dignified and respectful. This is followed by a lovely blessing at home by our vicar and a reception follows. The whole day is filled with laughter and joy. We shall always have this lovely memory to look back on and Christmas Eve will always be a special day.

In my life I am happy. I have achieved my ambition of becoming a therapist and being legally joined to Clare. My children have grown up with the usual problems that people have from time to time, but they are fine and living full happy lives. I have two wonderful grandchildren and a loving partner, not forgetting Misty, our dog, who brings laughter and pleasure into our lives.

Lightning Source UK Ltd.
Milton Keynes UK
UKHW041832170319
339331UK00001B/7/P